C000016309

Psychosocial Approaches

For Churchill Livingstone:

Commissioning Editor: Heidi Allen
Project Development Manager: Dinah Thom
Project Manager: Andrea Hill
Designer: Judith Wright

Psychosocial Approaches to Podiatry

A Companion for Practice

Anne Mandy

BSc(Hons) MSc PhD DPodM CertEd

Senior Research Fellow, Clinical Research Centre,
School of Health Professions, University of Brighton,
Eastbourne, UK

Kevin Lucas

BA DPhil PGDipHEd PGCAP HMFPHMed RMN RGN

Senior Lecturer in Psychology Applied to Healthcare,
Division of Physiotherapy, School of Health Professions,
University of Brighton, Eastbourne, UK

Janet McInnes

BSc(Hons) DPodM CertFEd

Principal Lecturer, Division of Podiatry,
School of Health Professions, University of Brighton,
Eastbourne, UK

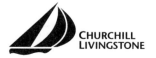

CHURCHILL
LIVINGSTONE

CHURCHILL LIVINGSTONE
An imprint of Elsevier Science Limited

© 2003, Elsevier Science Limited. All rights reserved.

The right of Anne Mandy, Kevin Lucas and Janet McInnes to be identified as authors of this work has been asserted by them in accordance with the Copyright, Designs and Patents Act 1988

No part of this publication may be reproduced, stored in a retrieval system, or transmitted in any form or by any means, electronic, mechanical, photocopying, recording or otherwise, without either the prior permission of the publishers (Permissions Manager, Elsevier Science Ltd, Robert Stevenson House, 1–3 Baxter's Place, Leith Walk, Edinburgh EH1 3AF), or a licence permitting restricted copying in the United Kingdom issued by the Copyright Licensing Agency, 90 Tottenham Court Road, London W1T 4LP.

First published 2003

ISBN 0 443 07156 X

British Library Cataloguing in Publication Data
A catalogue record for this book is available from the British Library

Library of Congress Cataloging in Publication Data
A catalog record for this book is available from the Library of Congress

Note
Medical knowledge is constantly changing. As new information becomes available, changes in treatment, procedures, equipment and the use of drugs become necessary. The authors and the publishers have taken care to ensure that the information given in this text is accurate and up to date. However, readers are strongly advised to confirm that the information, especially with regard to drug usage, complies with the latest legislation and standards of practice.

your source for books,
journals and multimedia
in the health sciences
www.elsevierhealth.com

The
publisher's
policy is to use
paper manufactured
from sustainable forests

Printed in China by RDC Group Limited

Contents

Preface **vii**

Introduction: using case-based learning **1**

1. Sociology of the podiatry profession **9**

2. Jenny Fraser – a newly qualified podiatrist **17**

3. David Humphries – private practitioners and continuous professional development **23**

4. Suzi Dalton – problems associated with middle age **27**

5. Charles Walters – problems of retirement and the sickness role **41**

6. James Watt – problems of personality and addictive behaviour **51**

7. Sheetal Joshi – a patient from an ethnic minority **61**

8. Enid Hilton – a recently bereaved elderly lady **67**

9. Bill Canning – the relationship between socioeconomic status and health **77**

10. Olivia Saunders – working with children and their parents **85**

11. Peter Brennan – dealing with sensitive and confidential material **93**

12. Harriet Edmondson – an adolescent with a suspected eating disorder **99**

13. Margaret Knowles – the conflict between medical and social needs **109**

14. Dorothy Atkins – the importance of self-efficacy **119**

15. Sophie Miller – a disabled adolescent with an interest in complementary medicine   **127**

16. George Archer – a person with diabetes who smokes   **137**

Glossary   **147**

Index   **155**

Preface

If one does not understand a person, one tends to regard him as a fool.

Carl Jung

In everyday clinical practice, podiatrists will encounter patients who have a range of problems that need to be understood. The aim of this book is to provide a problem- and case-based approach to understanding psychological and social difficulties that people often experience and present to practitioners. To our knowledge this is the first book of its kind for undergraduate podiatry students.

The clinical case studies and vignettes presented have been designed to meet a variety of needs. They will assist in preparing podiatry students and podiatrists intellectually and emotionally for situations encountered in practice. The book also attempts to empower clinicians to develop their clinical skills. The cases presented are based on real patients we have treated. Anonymized, they provide a vehicle for learning and illustrate the importance of understanding psychosocial issues in the context of holistic podiatric care. By contrast, the two podiatrists introduced in this book are entirely fictitious but possess characteristics that merit consideration.

This approach has determined the format in which the book is written: the main chapters are organized as individual patient case studies with relevant psychological theory attached. Attention is also given to social–psychological issues pertinent to both newly qualified and experienced podiatric practitioners. Theory is thus explained in the context of the presenting patient in a spirit of problem-based learning, enabling the reader to acquire knowledge and skills that would otherwise be gained more slowly. This book is designed to be an introduction to important applied psychology in clinical practice. Where a more extensive understanding of psychological theory is required, the reader is referred to appropriate sources. This volume is designed for self-directed learning but may also be used as a basis for action learning sets or informal discussion groups where cases will stimulate interest, dialogue and debate. Each section poses questions for the student to consider and provides an explanation of key issues. The learning activities and challenges will draw on theoretical models underpinning psychological theory. These are then applied to podiatry in a clinically useful way. At the end of each chapter there is a summary of important psychological theory, directed reading and references.

We would like to thank Dr Philip Mandy for his contribution to Chapter 1.

Anne Mandy
Kevin Lucas
Eastbourne 2003   Janet McInnes

Introduction: using case-based learning

Rabbit is clever. Rabbit has Brain. I suppose that is why he never understands anything.

A. A. Milne, *Winnie-the-Pooh*

Case-based learning is an educational strategy (Colliver 2000) in which the learner works in a self-directed manner towards the understanding or resolution of a practice-related issue. The learning process encourages reflective, critical and active learning and enhances the acquisition of clinical reasoning, critical thinking and judgement. Active learning empowers and inspires the learner by providing opportunities for success, achievement and enjoyment of learning.

The practice of podiatry is as much an art as a science. Each patient presents as a unique individual and multidimensional challenge that requires the podiatrist to have a cognitive model for clinical reasoning and professional skills (Cote 1993). Through the exploration of issues presented by the patients, the learner engages in the process of critical thinking while applying and integrating new information, and uses clinical reasoning to determine the best outcome for the patient. It is our intention that podiatry students using this book will embark on their education using a strategy that both results in a professional qualification and begins to develop a basis for lifelong learning, resulting in greater clinical success and satisfaction.

1

THE ROLE OF THE STUDENT

All students need to develop the professional skills and work habits of an autonomous professional clinician. This development results from experience in working with patients. The process of acquiring appropriate information and skills in order to undertake clinical reasoning and decision making is multifactorial and complex and for some students this transition is difficult to make. Students and therapists need to be able to apply appropriate theory in the context of complex situations with the added constraints of the realities of clinical practice. The patient scenarios contained within this text require the student to consider the issues presented by the characters in order to have an improved understanding of the patient's needs.

Each section begins with a summary of information describing the content of the case. A clinical podiatric presentation for each character is then provided for the student to consider.

The characters in this book are based on patients drawn from the authors' own professional practice. Changes have been made in order to protect their identities.

HEALTH PSYCHOLOGY AND THE PODIATRY STUDENT

Until the last decade, much of the curriculum for podiatry students was concerned with the scientific and theoretical basis for clinical work. Theories underpinning patient behaviour were largely ignored in the belief that exposure to clinical experience would suffice. This 'medical model' has had an enormous influence over podiatric education and practice. The model demands a mechanistic approach, regarding the symptoms of illness as the failure of an anatomical structure or of a system. Health and disease are also considered to be contrasting states and are thus defined solely in mechanistic terms. In these terms, 'health' is exemplified by the body being in good working order, while any deviation from the norm is seen as disease. In the view of the medical model, treatment is provided to restore physiological function or to remove faulty structures.

Engel (1977) proposed a biopsychosocial model of health, suggesting that, while pathogens may be responsible for changing health status, behavioural, psychological and social influences have an equally powerful effect on a person's state of health or illness. In addition, recovery from illness is now known to be strongly mediated by psychosocial factors such as personality, coping styles and psychological wellbeing. It is also now well-established that an individual's environment and social networks fundamentally influence health status, prognosis in the case of disease and life expectancy.

Students in podiatry must learn to appreciate the complexity of patients' needs, which are beyond the simple pathology that instigates their arrival at the clinic.

While we all have a general understanding of the terms 'illness' and 'disease', it is important to have a common understanding of these terms for the purposes of this book. Our definition of illness is rooted as much in the individual's experience of being unwell as in the pathological state of an organ or system. Moreover, it is important to recognize that it is common for a patient to have a disease without experiencing illness, for example in some preclinical cancers. Conversely, it is possible for a patient to experience illness in the absence of organic pathology, for example in anxiety states or depression.

In recent years, health psychology has addressed many aspects of the experience of illness and distress, such as pain, addiction and bereavement. Some podiatry students may encounter these experiences in their own lives but not all podiatry students will have done so at the time they begin their professional training. It is therefore important that they appreciate the magnitude of the impact such factors have on their patients, and it is this appreciation that is the aim of this book.

The relationship between any practitioner and patient depends on many factors, including gender, age, culture, social class and the nature of the therapeutic interaction. The nature of the therapeutic interaction in turn varies according to the professional discipline. The relationship between podiatrists and their patients is in some ways rather different from that associated with other disciplines. Firstly, the time that podiatrists spend with their patients on a one-to-one basis is frequently longer than that of other professionals. This often results in patients using the podiatrist as a 'confidante'.

Secondly, the podiatric patients rarely present for treatment because of serious or life-threatening illness. Podiatric patients usually have considerable understanding of their condition and may well have experienced it for a protracted period of time. The quality of the professional–patient relationship is thus much more equal than in many other settings.

However, the clinical environment in which podiatrists practise is not always conducive to accommodating some of the patient's psychological needs. The clinical layout of the practice and the use of surgical instruments, and podiatric treatments is reminiscent of that of dentists, and certainly not an ideal environment in which to develop a therapeutic relationship. The clinical environment and nature of podiatric practice may particularly affect new patients. New patients are exposed to a range of unusual sights, noises, smells and procedures, which may make them feel anxious. The podiatrist should always endeavour to put patients at their ease, explain carefully what they should expect from the consultation and use minimal intervention where possible. When designing clinical environments, efforts to 'humanize' what may appear to be a cold and sterile surgery are likely to be much appreciated by patients. Similarly, the podiatrist should be aware that the conventional position adopted for treatment (with the podiatrist seated at the patient's feet) is not ideal for interviewing and history taking, during which maintaining eye contact is of considerable importance. However, most patients become familiar and comfortable with the environment after the initial visit.

Podiatrists work in a range of environments, including as part of the National Health Service, in private practice, through commercial high-street companies, in occupational health departments, as well as in education and research. While such variety offers many opportunities to achieve job satisfaction, some research suggests that the need for collegiality and identified roles within teams is the key to its realization (Mandy 2000). These issues are explored further in a later chapter.

INTRODUCTION TO THE CASE STUDIES

The characters presented within this book are based on real people. While it is unlikely that any one podiatrist's case load would contain patients with such a complex range of problems at any one time, the characters are used as a vehicle to illustrate a range of issues that most podiatrists will encounter at some time during the course of their professional lives. It is not the aim of this book to make all podiatrists into quasi-psychologists. Its aim is to introduce the student to some important psychological concepts that may influence and improve their clinical practice and provide the clinician-in-training with skills that will enhance clinical reasoning by better understanding their patients' needs.

In the early stages of a professional life, newly qualified practitioners may spend much of their time developing clinical skills in order to be able to cope with the demands of professional practice. At this stage this 'clinical companion' will help to explain some of the feelings that practitioners may experience. The character of *Jenny Fraser* identifies some of the issues associated with a new podiatry job, including sources of occupational stress and ways in which she can deal effectively with her new situation. *David Humphries*, on the other hand, presents issues pertinent to practitioners who have been working in practice for some time. The chapter explores the autonomous nature of private practice and the increasing need of practitioners to undertake continuous professional development. Both these practitioners will have to consider their professional development needs.

The scenarios described in this book have been carefully constructed in order to introduce the student to patients experiencing a range of life events. Appropriate psychological and sociological theory is provided and illustrated in the context of the characters.

Olivia Saunders presents an interesting challenge for the podiatrist who is involved in a complex interaction involving a child and her parents. The importance of good interpersonal and communication skills is highlighted and the need for appropriate health promotion approaches is also discussed. *Harriet Edmondson* is an equally complex character who displays some of the difficulties faced by contemporary adolescents. Issues of professional boundaries are considered. *Sophie Miller* is an adolescent who suffers from a serious physical disability. She is disillusioned with conventional medicine and seeks alternatives. She is not understood by her family, who are unable to support her. The chapter discusses some of the typical concerns of adolescence.

The aspirations and frustrations of a young executive are explored in the character of *James Watt*. James is a product of his times; he is competitive, materialistic and intolerant of having his chosen lifestyle frustrated. The chapter explores the psychology of personality, addictive and aggressive behaviours and the psychological responses to pain.

Suzi Dalton exhibits some of the problems that can be associated with middle age and the menopause. In addition she exemplifies some of the insecurities and vulnerability that are commonplace in contemporary British society. Psychological factors addressed are the Health Belief Model, the menopause, self-esteem and the therapeutic relationship.

Charles Walters and *Dorothy Atkins* are facing some of the challenges posed by the retirement years. Taken together they provide a contrast that clearly demonstrates the crucial contribution that social support makes to health and wellbeing. The theory of reasoned action is used to explain how Charles makes decisions about his health. The sick role, self-help groups and retirement are also discussed. The character of Dorothy is used to highlight the importance of positive traits, the positive effect that family and social ties can have on illness, self-efficacy, control and optimism. *Enid Hilton* is experiencing bereavement. The processes she goes through as a result are an essential part of the understanding of all healthcare professionals, particularly those who deal predominantly with older people.

The importance of confidentiality in professional practice is emphasized by the character of *Peter Brennan*, where the need to understand professional boundaries and competencies is explored in relation to his HIV status. A sensitivity to cultural differences is essential to podiatric practice and the character of *Sheetal Joshi* explores this need in detail. The complications of language differences and working through interpreters is also considered.

The influence of socioeconomic status on health is illustrated in the cases of *Bill Canning*. Bill is disempowered by his 'better off' associates and his health-related behaviour is mediated by social exclusion. The character of *George Archer* is used to illustrate current psychological theory in relation to decision-making processes and substance use.

Margaret Knowles, like all of the characters in this book, is based upon a real person. Her story clearly portrays the sacrifices that people are prepared to make in order to meet the needs of others rather than their own. Understanding the motivations and values of patients is necessary in order to understand their behaviour. In Margaret's case her attachment to her family was overwhelmingly more important to her than her own welfare, with tragic consequences.

Clearly as the podiatrist's clinical and life experiences expand, so too will her/his abilities and confidence to work with a wide range of patients grow. Developing an understanding of psychosocial issues in relation to patients will not only improve the care that s/he can offer but will also result in a more rewarding and satisfying career. This aspect of professional practice will continue to grow long after the podiatrist's clinical skills have reached a point of excellence.

The psychological theory expounded in this book will serve as an aid to your clinical practice. Understanding the principles outlined in each chapter will help you to deal more effectively with a wide range of patients and their problems. However, this book cannot be a substitute for important qualities that you must learn to develop for yourself. Warmth, empathy and human understanding cannot be taught in a classroom or seminar, or by reading a book. They are, however, the very attributes that will distinguish an adequate technician from a true practitioner.

REFERENCES

Colliver JA 2000 Effectiveness of problem-based learning curricula: research and theory. Academic Medicine 75, 259–266

Cote M 1993 Case method case teaching and the making of a manager. In Klein HE (ed) Case method and application: innovation through co-operation. World Association for Case Method Research and Application, Needham

Engel G 1977 The need for a new medical model: a challenge for biomedicine. Science 196, 126–129

Mandy A 2000 Burnout and work stress in newly qualified podiatrists working in the NHS. British Journal of Podiatry and Chiropody May 32, 31–34

1

Sociology of the podiatry profession

The aim of this chapter is to provide a brief sociological perspective of podiatry, and of its associated implications for podiatric practice.

SIMILARITIES BETWEEN PODIATRY AND MEDICINE

An interprofessional hierarchy has long been recognized within medicine. Merton et al (1956), Becker et al (1961) and Schartzbaum et al (1973) have all described such a hierarchy, led by specialist surgery, followed by general surgery and thereafter by various divisions of internal medicine. General practice and dermatology follow, with psychiatry generally being regarded as the least prestigious branch of the profession (Abbott 1981). Within the healthcare professions, a hierarchy has begun to develop that closely mirrors that found in medicine. For example, podiatric surgery has an extensive history but has only recently developed into a speciality in its own right. Borthwick (2000) describes the issue of podiatric surgery and the boundaries of clinical practice. The training to become a podiatric surgeon requires postgraduate study and clinical practice in order to meet the requirements of the Faculty of Podiatric Surgery. Similarly, there are emergent specialisms in podiatric medicine, including rheumatology, diabetic care, paediatrics and biomechanics. Observation suggests that those podiatrists who specialize are deemed to be higher in the professional hierarchy than are those who remain generalists. It may be salutary to note that, by contrast, there is as yet no 'speciality' for the podiatric care of the elderly, despite the fact that older people represent the majority of our patients.

9

PODIATRY AND OTHER HEALTH PROFESSIONS

In general, podiatry as a profession has had a long and convoluted history. It was solely in search of recognition (and hence status) that a few of the many bodies formerly representing podiatrists came together under the Board of Registration of Medical Auxiliaries (BRMA) recognition in 1942. It was not until 18 years later that a 1960 Act of Parliament established the Council for Professions Supplementary to Medicine (CPSM) as the statutory and regulatory body for these professions. Each professional discipline within the Council was then given its own regulatory Board.

The Health Professions Council (HPC) replaced the CPSM in April 2002, and there are no longer separate boards for each profession. Within the HPC, interdisciplinary hierarchies are still seen to exist. Yet as the professions concerned are roughly comparable in terms of income, power and education, such hierarchies cannot be explained by traditional criteria.

Early sociologists have employed a number of approaches in attempts to explain the process of professionalization; these theoretical orientations are outside the scope of this book but are described in considerable detail elsewhere (Carr-Saunders & Wilson 1933, Parsons 1939). Later, Greenwood (1957) considered the successive steps any occupation goes through in order to achieve professional status. He suggests that the process involves the following steps:

1. People begin doing (full-time) something that needs to be done. The sick were always nursed but technical and organizational developments created nursing as a profession.

2. Early practitioners (or the public) campaign for the establishment of a formal training school. While not all schools originated in universities (e.g. in the case of public sector administrators, city planners and accountants), they all eventually sought support from universities.

3. Proponents of prescribed training, and the first alumni, combine to form a professional association.

4. Pressure is exerted in order to win legal protection of the job territory and its sustaining code of ethics.

Eventually, rules are made to eliminate the unqualified, to reduce internal competition and to protect clients. The ideal of service then becomes embodied in a formal code of ethics (Wilensky 1964). More recently, Storch & Stinson (1988) have suggested that the two main distinguishing characteristics of a profession are a body of abstract knowledge and an ideal of service.

PROFESSIONALISM AND PROFESSIONAL STATUS

While status differences create gross hierarchical structures, they do not automatically produce the exact *order* of hierarchy, which is generated by measures of honour, power, wealth and knowledge. Abbott (1981) maintains that income, power and client status are important factors in determining such order. Yet income may be an unreliable determinant of status; for example, within NHS medicine, salaries are similar irrespective of the area of specialism yet different specialisms clearly have different status.

However, Abbott also suggests complexity as an alternative basis for determining interprofessional status; put simply, high status is attributed to non-routine work. General practitioners refer difficult, non-routine cases to specialists, who handle them or in turn pass them on to even more specialist practitioners. Conversely, routine aspects of professional practice are often delegated to the para-professional level (Freidson 1970). In the case of podiatry, patients may be referred 'upwards' to specialist podiatric surgeons or 'downwards' to foot-care assistants.

Most foot conditions worsen with age, and systemic complications are more likely in the elderly. It is therefore the case that the majority of patients in receipt of podiatry care are over 50 years of age. Many authors have noted the ageism intrinsic to Western society. Given the current status of podiatry in relation to other health professions, Abbott may be correct in citing client status as an indicator of professional status. If this the case, then podiatric practitioners must develop not only their own professional status but also coping mechanisms for dealing with the attitudes of other professionals in the meantime.

Education and knowledge have always been emphasized by professions seeking higher status (Larson 1977). Abbott (1981) maintains that 'the overall correlation of education and social status is undeniable'. However, this fails to explain the relative status of professional groups whose education and levels of knowledge may be similar, for example podiatrists and physiotherapists. Even though both receive education of a similar level (in some institutions physiotherapy and podiatry students share classes), the British public perceives physiotherapists as being of higher status than podiatrists (Mandy 2000).

Two other factors may also influence the status of a professional group: the gender balance of the profession and the nature of the professional practice. Professions having a higher proportion of women members consistently have lower status than professions that are male-dominated. A frequently cited example is the relationship of nursing to medicine. However, medical school intakes in the UK have been balanced by gender for many years, and certain areas of nursing (notably psychiatric nursing) have always attracted roughly equal numbers of men and women. Nevertheless, in both professions women are under-represented in senior positions. Thus Abbott's fourth factor, the nature of professional activity, may provide better explanations of the hierarchical structure of the health professions. However, it is this factor that is by far the least investigated.

PROFESSIONAL AUTONOMY

For a paramedical profession to attain autonomy, it must concern itself with a discrete area of work that can be separated from the main body of medicine. It must also be able to practise that area of work without routine contact with, or dependence on, doctors. From an early period, podiatry has provided services through an occupational structure separate from medicine. This is also true of opticians, speech therapists and speech pathologists. But despite gaining relative autonomy of practice, higher status has not yet followed.

Monopolization is an established tactic for restricting the number of competitors and ensuring the maintenance of a profession.

Dentists gained such a monopoly with professional closure in 1921, despite continued conflict with medicine. At the time of writing, podiatry has still to acquire any such legal privileges. A profession maintains its position by recognizing that changes in medical knowledge and technology, as well as changing patterns of morbidity and mortality, result in important modifications (Elton 1977). Some roles become obsolete, others emerge: specialization breeds occupational homogeneity and groups with conflicting interests appear, thus weakening professional solidarity and potentially threatening the profession's dominant position. External challenges come from different sources: other occupations, whether they are in direct competition or in a position of subordination to the dominant group, also try to improve their status and increase their work autonomy.

Historically, dominant professions such as medicine and law have experienced inter- and intraprofessional conflicts as well as conflict with the state. Their responses have involved both their clientele and the recruitment of 'suitable' new members in the maintenance of occupational cohesiveness, a process that has been described as 'patrolling the entrance gate'. In organizing formal training and in instituting qualifying procedures, occupations seeking professional status assert that only their members have the competence to perform certain tasks or to deliver certain services. Finally, professional groups engage in political activity to gain state recognition and to develop a legal monopoly of certain activities.

PRACTITIONER–PATIENT RELATIONSHIPS

In considering the nature of practice it is important to consider the relationship between the professional and the patient. Parsons (1951) portrayed the doctor–patient relationship as one of reciprocity, in which the doctor and patient have certain obligations and privileges attached to their respective roles. Morgan et al (1985) suggest that Parsons's analysis of the relationship is based on the two parties being socialized in their roles. The patient, as part of the obligations attached to the sick role, is expected to seek technically competent help, usually from a doctor, to trust the doctor and to accept that the doctor is a competent help-giver. Conversely, the doctor is expected:

- to act in accordance with the health needs of his or her patient;
- to follow the rules of professional conduct;
- to use a high degree of expertise and knowledge;
- to remain objective and emotionally neutral.

This reciprocity is particularly pertinent to the case of *Charles Walters*, a patient described in Chapter 5.

A more detailed analysis of the doctor–patient relationship was developed by Szasz & Hollender (1956) and it is considered in greater detail in Chapter 4.

The practitioner–patient relationship will be explored later in the book in the context of the character of *Suzi Dalton* in Chapter 4.

Podiatry patients are often prepared to assume an active role in their treatment. Freidson (1970) presented patients as active and critical in rejecting professional services when they contradicted their own conceptions of illness. In some cases, he argued, patients perceived their own and other lay alternatives to be superior to professional medical opinion. When examining podiatric care it is interesting to consider these issues. Patients are able to observe the whole process of treatment of their feet and indeed, often attempt their own treatment, sometimes with painful or damaging results. They have a clear idea of both what they think they require and how it should be achieved. Because of their ability to observe the podiatrist at work they can take an active role in their own treatment. Thus Freidson's analysis may be applied accurately to podiatry. Clinicians are advised to consider carefully the patient's social and cultural context. The character of *Sheetal Joshi* (Chapter 7) considers this issue in greater detail.

People are able to examine their own feet. As a result, patients attending podiatric services will have formed a view of the aetiology of their condition and will attend for treatment rather than preventative monitoring. Monitoring is an important part of podiatric care, particularly for patients suffering from diabetes. Such patients often experience complications such as peripheral arterial disease and its associated neuropathy. Minor cuts or abrasions, if untreated, may result in ulceration and ultimately in amputation of the toes or limb. In addition, regular monitoring of the vascular status of the patient may identify such complications early enough to initiate treatment that will minimize their effects. These issues will be discussed further in the characters of *George Archer* in Chapter 16 and *Charles Walters* in Chapter 5.

Such monitoring requires well-developed communication skills on the part of the podiatrist. Communication skills and communication theory are discussed in the context of the characters *Suzi Dalton* in Chapter 4, *Enid Hilton* in Chapter 8 and *James Watt* in Chapter 6.

Professionalization is pertinent to podiatry practice, where the desire to improve professional status may be in danger of overshadowing the intrinsic altruism of the occupation. Perhaps ironically, there is no evidence that an increase in professional status improves the practitioner's self-esteem or feelings of professional worth. Traditionally high-status professionals may also suffer from low self-esteem, and the prevalence of psychological problems among 'higher' professionals has reached alarming proportions. Nevertheless, social status has profound effects upon human relationships, and this issue is discussed in the context of the character *Bill Canning* in Chapter 9. Podiatry currently has comparatively low professional status, partly because it does not meet some established status criteria but mainly because much of its work can be routine and less than glamorous. However, this should not deter its practitioners: if podiatrists take an objective view of their own position and accept the reality that expert foot care is, and increasingly will be required, then the profession could prosper. Paradoxically, not by attempting to pursue the criteria for achieving high status but by establishing its own professional niche and improving its own expertise, the standing of the profession could rise.

FURTHER READING

Johnson TJ 1972 Professions and power. Macmillan, London
Radley A 1994 Making sense of illness. Sage, London
Turner BS 1995 Medical power and social knowledge. Sage, London

REFERENCES

Abbott A 1981 Status and status strain in the professions. American Journal of Sociology 86, 819–835

Becker HS, Geer B, Hughes EC, Strauss AL 1961 Boys in white. Chicago University Press, Chicago, IL

Borthwick AM 2000 Challenging medicine: the case of podiatric surgery, work employment and society. British Journal of Podiatry 14, 369–383

Carr-Saunders AM, Wilson PA 1933 The professions. Clarendon Press, Oxford

Elton MA 1977 Medical autonomy: challenge and response. In Bernard K, Lee K (ed) Conflicts in the National Health Service. Croom Helm, London

Freidson E 1970 Profession of medicine. Dodd Mead & Co, New York

Greenwood E 1957 Attributes of a profession. Social Work 2, 44–55

Larson MS 1977 The rise of professionalism. University of California Press, CA

Mandy P 2000 The nature and status of chiropody and dentistry. DPhil thesis, University of Sussex

Merton RK, Bloom S, Rogoff N 1956 Columbia Pennsylvania studies in the sociology of medical education. Journal of Medical Education 31, 552–565

Morgan M, Calnan M, Manning N 1985 Sociological approaches to health and medicine. Croom Helm, London

Parsons T 1939 The professions and social structure. In Essays in sociological theory. Free Press, New York

Parsons T 1951 The social system. Free Press, Glencoe, IL

Schartzbaum A, McGrath J, Rothman R 1973 The perception of prestige differences amongst medical specialities. Social Science and Medicine 7, 365–371

Storch J, Stinson S 1988 Concepts of deprofessionalisation with application to nursing. In White R (ed) Politics in nursing: past present and future, vol 3. John Wiley, Chichester

Szasz TS, Hollender MH 1956 A contribution to the philosophy of medicine. Archives of Internal Medicine 97, 585–592

Wilensky HL 1964 The professionalisation of everyone. American Journal of Sociology 70, 137–158

2

Jenny Fraser – a newly qualified podiatrist

Far and away the best prize that life offers is the chance to work hard at work worth doing.

Theodore Roosevelt

Jenny is a newly qualified podiatrist who graduated from university last summer. She is an enthusiastic and cheerful young woman who always wanted to be a podiatrist and is thrilled at the prospect of commencing her new career. She has recently taken up her first post as a junior podiatrist working for the state health provider. Jenny has returned to her parents' home after a period of 3 years at university. She is finding the constraints of home life difficult after her independence as a student. She is also having to build a new social life because most of her school friends also went away to university and have not returned.

FACTORS INFLUENCING JENNY

Jenny chose to take up employment near home principally because she has a large student loan that she has to repay. Jenny was particularly attracted to her current job because of the variety of work offered and the range of experiences she would encounter. The job includes community, hospital, domiciliary and some administrative duties.

However, on some days of the week Jenny has to travel between clinic sites that are some distance apart, and this often involves her missing her lunch break. Jenny is thoroughly enjoying her job but finds the amount of paperwork and administration involved irritating and excessive. She was not anticipating this aspect of the work, and finds it an unexpected burden. She is uncertain why she has to complete certain tasks and what happens to the information that she collects. She finds that in trying to keep up with all the administration and paperwork she often runs late with her patients' appointments and by the end of the day she is quite behind schedule. One of the consequences of running late is that some of the patients become irritated and demanding, which causes Jenny to become anxious and frustrated.

The environment in which Jenny now works is very different to that of the university. She no longer works alongside friends and colleagues and finds working in single-chair clinics lonely. The only contact she has with her professional colleagues is on the two afternoons a month when she works in the orthotics laboratory. The reception and ancillary staff who support her clinical work at the various sites are all extraordinarily warm and helpful. However, Jenny misses the professional discussion, support and friendship she had while at university. These difficulties are inevitably exacerbated when trying to help certain patients. This is illustrated in the cases of *James Watt* (Chapter 6) and *Margaret Knowles* (Chapter 13).

In the case of *James Watt*, Jenny needs to learn how to deal with patients who are aggressive and demanding without becoming upset herself. Much of the resilience necessary to achieve this may be acquired through good communication skills and skilled patient management. In the case of *Margaret Knowles*, it is essential for Jenny to be able to set treatment objectives that meet Margaret's needs at the time of presentation.

The Podiatry Department is also undergoing a period of reorganization and staff change. There are currently two members of staff on maternity leave and one unfilled vacancy. Efficiency savings are being enforced and the podiatry budget is currently slightly overspent. While not being paid as a senior II, Jenny has been asked to take on the duties usually performed by more senior colleagues.

Challenge 1: Identify the likely sources of stress for Jenny in her new job

Workload and time pressures are strongly correlated with emotional exhaustion and burnout (Lee & Ashforth 1996). A study of newly qualified podiatrists in the UK (Mandy 2000) further supported this finding. The early post-qualification period is a challenging time when professional, time management and general organizational skills are being developed. There are several ways in which work can be stressful.

These include organizational problems such as insufficient back-up, long or unsociable hours, poor status, low pay and limited promotion prospects, uncertainty and insecurity of employment. Moreover, issues such as unclear role specifications, role conflict, unrealistically high self-expectations (perfectionism), inability to influence decision making, frequent clashes with superiors, isolation from colleague support, lack of variety, poor communication, inadequate leadership, conflicts with colleagues, inability to finish a job and fighting unnecessary battles may also contribute to stress at work.

Lack of control over work has been identified as a source of stress that may lead to poor health. Many studies have found that heavy job demand and low control, or decreased decision freedom, lead to job dissatisfaction, mental strain and cardiovascular disease (Sutton & Kahn 1984, Sauter et al 1989).

Research has found that participating actively in the planning and execution of work tasks reduces stress and hence improves health status (Israel et al 1989). A study by Jackson (1983) found that simple attendance at staff meetings (non-active participation) did not of itself influence perceived job stress. However, those people who participated actively in staff meetings reported lower job stress, improved job satisfaction and lower absenteeism. Similarly, Israel et al (1989) concluded that the ability to control or influence work factors is linked to the incidence of cardiovascular disease and to psychosomatic disorders, depression and job dissatisfaction.

Role conflict can exist in many forms. There may be conflict between the job and the employee's personal values. Roles that are not clearly defined are termed ambiguous and are a source of conflict that is associated with lower productivity, increased tension, dissatisfaction and work stress (Lindquist & Whitehead 1986).

Every podiatry department will have a slightly different induction process and period, ranging from the very simple brief explanation of health and safety procedures to a 6-month induction. In the most supportive departments, new members of staff are gradually introduced to all aspects of the job within the institution. The advantages of continued support, supervision and mentoring of staff at all levels is now widely acknowledged.

In addition, most professional codes of practice contain an expectation that staff should practise within ethical guidelines, making it essential to be able to voice concerns about patient care and patient services. In order for this to be possible, professionals need to develop confidence and assertiveness.

Effective time management requires the ability to cope with all elements of the job within a specified time. Time management includes clarification of job responsibilities, duties and roles followed by appropriate allocation of time to each of these components. Skills may then be developed in prioritizing, planning and delegation.

Prioritizing work also ensures that important issues are addressed first. Identification of 'time robbers' such as unnecessary meetings and phone calls will reduce wasted time.

Challenge 2: What strategies can Jenny employ to ensure that she remains optimistic and healthy within her job?

Some of Jenny's friends from university work in a neighbouring health authority. At a recent reunion they reported very different experiences to Jenny's. Most of them have experienced an extensive induction programme and have been allocated a mentor who is an experienced practitioner. There is an organized programme of staff meetings, a programme of continuous professional development and various courses available for staff. A new scheme for clinical supervision is being developed by the entire staff team, which is aimed at providing mutual support. The exposure of this contrasting situation offers Jenny a different and more positive perspective on employment.

Lazarus (1991) has identified at least two strategies for reducing work-related stress:

• Alter the working conditions so that they are less stressful or more conducive to effective coping. This strategy is most appropriate for large numbers of workers working under severe conditions. Examples include altering physical annoyances such as noise levels, or changing organizational decision-making processes to include employees. In Jenny's case it is important that she is encouraged to contribute her opinions and suggestions at staff meetings and that, where possible, she is involved in teamwork.

• Make help available to employees to enable them to acquire more effective coping strategies for situations that are impossible or difficult to change.

SUMMARY

In order for Jenny to enjoy her job she must maintain a healthy balance between her work and her social life. Many individuals find that their social life is closely associated with their professional life and there are many special-interest groups in podiatry in which Jenny could meet colleagues with similar interests. Developing a programme of continuous professional development will also contribute significantly to her job satisfaction.

REFERENCES

Israel BA, House JS, Schurman SJ et al 1989 The relation of personal resources, participation, influence, interpersonal relationships and coping strategies to occupational stress, job strains and health: a multivariate analysis. Work Stress 3, 163–194

Jackson SE 1983 Participation in decision making as a strategy for reducing job-related strain. Journal of Applied Psychology 68, 3–19

Lazarus R 1991 Psychological stress in the workplace. Journal of Social Behaviour and Personality 6, 1–13

Lee RT Ashforth BE 1996 A meta analytic examination of the correlates of the three dimensions of job burnout. Journal of Applied Psychology 81, 123–133

Lindquist CA Whitehead JT 1986 Burnout, job stress and job satisfaction among southern correctional officers: perceptions and casual factors. Journal of Offender Counselling Services and Rehabilitation 10, 5–26

Mandy A 2000 Burnout and work stress in newly qualified podiatrists in the NHS. British Journal of Podiatry 3, 31–34

Sauter, S Hurrell J Jr, Cooper C 1989 Job control and worker health. John Wiley, New York

Sutton R, Kahn RL 1984 Prediction, understanding, and control as antidotes to organizational stress. In Lorsch J (ed) Handbook of organizational behavior. Harvard University Press, Cambridge, MA

3

David Humphries – private practitioners and continuous professional development

Loyalty to petrified opinions never yet broke a chain or freed a human soul in this world – and never will.

Mark Twain

David qualified as a chiropodist 20 years ago before the introduction of a degree in podiatry. He trained at a small college and lived at home during his period as a student. After qualifying, he bought an established practice from a retiring practitioner, in which he still works. In the last 10 years he has purchased one other practice in the next village and employs two part-time practitioners and a part-time receptionist. David is married to Betty, who, following some nursing experience, retrained as a foot-care assistant and works in his practice, where she also acts as receptionist.

David provides what he describes as 'a good traditional service', providing patients with 'what they want'. He has a busy caseload of patients who require regular appointments. David also has a large domiciliary caseload, which takes up two days of his week. Since qualifying, he has attended orthotics courses and has undertaken a course in small business management at a local further education college. David has not been able to find time to study for a degree in podiatry, as he is very committed to charitable work locally. His practice is successful and he is rewarded by the recommendation of his patients and by the high esteem in which he is held by the local business community. Until recently, there seemed little imperative to take his studies further. However, just recently he has noticed that the professional journal has been publishing articles about continuous professional development (CPD). Initially he thought this was directed towards those practitioners who had a degree. It is now clear to him from his local branch that the Society of Chiropodists and Podiatrists endorses CPD for all podiatrists. Members of the society are expected to accumulate a number of credits each year and to maintain a portfolio of CPD activity. Professional indemnity is linked to membership of the Society and thus this is of concern to David.

David finds this requirement daunting and remains to be convinced that such a development is entirely necessary or, indeed, that CPD should be compulsory. However, just recently one of his part-time staff has suggested that they introduce a sports injuries and biomechanics service. This would require David to learn new skills.

The nature of private practice is very different from that of health service practice. The relationship that develops between private practitioners and their patients can be long-standing, and friendships often result. The model of the practitioner–patient relationship proposed by Szasz & Hollender (1956; see Chapter 4) and also Parsons's sick role theory do not necessarily apply in private practice. Parsons (1951) suggests a set of rights and obligations for both practitioner and patient. Critics later questioned this theory because it does not explain the circumstances of chronic illness. The relationship that develops in private practice is akin to Szasz & Hollender's typology of mutual participation. Such a typology implies that the patient has a degree of power in the relationship and therefore takes responsibility for his/her own health. This is particularly pertinent in the case of private practice, where patients *choose* their practitioner and will only continue to consult them as long as they feel that their needs are being met.

David is an autonomous practitioner and is in complete control of his working environment. He is confident, experienced and makes all the decisions regarding his business. He does, however, consult his employees regarding their work practices and endeavours to be flexible and supportive of his two part-time colleagues. David is very accustomed to being in control of his life and is both anxious about and slightly affronted by the prospect of compulsory CPD. However, he realizes that part of his anxiety stems from a lack of confidence in his readiness to resume study and his fear of failure.

Nevertheless, the range of patients now seen in podiatry practice has changed since David trained, and this change in case-mix is likely to present David with a number of difficult problems. For example, it is unlikely that David will have encountered a patient such as *Harriet Edmondson* (Chapter 12). In addition to her psychological difficulties, Harriet is an adolescent who is likely to be demanding in ways that David will find difficult to manage. Similarly, *Peter Brennan* (Chapter 11) is likely to present David with issues that may challenge his personal beliefs.

The majority of patients attend a podiatrist for diagnosis and alleviation of their symptoms. In certain circumstances it may not be possible to offer a cure. Patients may also seek podiatric treatment and advice for symptoms resulting from systemic illness.

Furthermore, the professional role and provision of treatment is different in private practice from practice in the state sector. Private practitioners treat anyone who seeks their services. By contrast, NHS practitioners may be limited by local policies and may only treat patients who meet specific access criteria and who may thus present with more complex or severe conditions.

Challenge 1: Why is David reluctant to participate in continuous professional development?

David is currently feeling threatened for two reasons. The prospect of having to undertake CPD worries David because of the time required and because of the time that has elapsed since he last undertook any kind of formal study. Secondly, he feels inadequately prepared to provide a biomechanics service, as this is currently outside his scope of practice. Currently, David is avoiding addressing these issues. His habitual coping style is to ignore problems that make him feel uncomfortable or threatened rather than to address them directly.

Challenge 2: How could you avoid finding yourself in David's position?

As an undergraduate student you have many advantages over David. For example, you will learn to develop your critical analysis skills and to understand research methodology. These skills will enable you to keep abreast of developments in professional practice and to employ evidence-based practice. To do this effectively, it is essential for you to understand your own learning needs and to seek appropriate post-registration education. Your local branch of the Society of Chiropodists and Podiatrists offers CPD advice.

REFERENCES

Parsons T 1951 The social system. Free Press, Glencoe, IL
Szasz TS, Hollender MH 1956 A contribution to the philosophy of medicine. Archives of Internal Medicine 97, 585–592

4

Suzi Dalton – problems associated with middle age

A serious mention of menopause is usually met with uneasy silence; a sneering reference to it is usually met with relieved sniggers. Both the silence and the sniggering are pretty sure indications of taboo.

Ursula K. Le Guin

Suzi is a slim, attractive woman who works as an air hostess for a large international airline. She is 48 years old but looks slightly older than her years. She has been an air hostess since she left school and has thoroughly enjoyed the glamorous lifestyle offered by international travel. Just recently, she has begun to find it more difficult to cope with long-haul flights, and finds herself more tired than previously. She jokes that 'Life begins at 40' but is privately concerned about her changed appearance and worries about the recent irregularity of her menstrual cycle. She reports feeling more stressed than usual and 'wound up inside'. Suzi finds herself relying more heavily on cigarettes to help get her through the difficult times. She has never had a weight problem. However, recently she has noticed that her waist is not as slim as it used to be. Although loath to admit it, she feels that her job was easier when she was younger, and she had more fun.

Suzi was divorced a year ago after her husband left her for a younger woman. Her manner is brusque and there is a hint of aggression in her voice. There has been an error in her appointment date and time, and she has been unpleasant and patronizing to the receptionist.

PODIATRIC PRESENTATION

Suzi presents with painful lesser toes and a painful first meta-tarsophalangeal joint (hallux valgus or bunion). She reports that the pain is so severe that it prevents her from walking comfortably and is affecting her work. On examination, she has deformed toes with a number of soft tissue lesions. Some of these are very inflamed and may be infected. In addition, there are areas of hard skin on the soles and heels of both feet. She wears high-heeled court shoes for both work and leisure; her work shoes are part of her uniform.

FACTORS THAT INFLUENCE SUZI'S BEHAVIOUR

Suzi believes she must remain youthful in appearance in order to satisfy her employer's expectations. However, she is beginning to notice the signs of the ageing process, which causes her concern. Her tolerance to stress is reduced and she finds she is starting to smoke more.

Suzi has low self-esteem, which may be associated with her physical appearance, which is very important to her. The slight increase in weight she has noticed is of great concern. In addition, her recent divorce has left her with feelings of rejection and inadequacy, which contributes to her reduced self-esteem. Divorce is a life event that is associated with high levels of stress. In the post-divorce period, people can experience symptoms similar to those who have been bereaved. Suzi's aggression may stem from her low self-esteem, her hormonal changes and her general unhappiness.

A number of social–psychological models have been proposed in attempts to explain people's health-related behaviours. One such model that has been very influential in healthcare is known as the Health Belief Model (Becker & Rosenstock 1984). This model is summarized in Figure 4.1.

The major components of the model are as follows:

- **Demographic factors** – Suzi's beliefs are influenced by her age, gender and occupation. She works in an industry in which physical appearance, youth and attractiveness are considered to be important attributes.

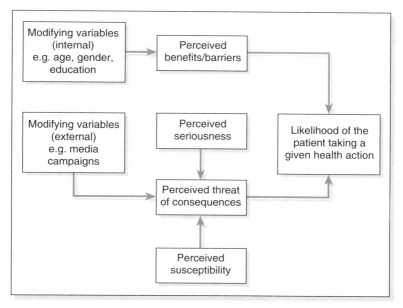

Fig. 4.1   The Health Belief Model (based on Becker & Rosenstock 1984)

- **Susceptibility** – The likelihood of an individual performing any given behaviour is in part determined by how susceptible they believe they are to any outcomes that may be associated with that behaviour. In Suzi's case, the likelihood of her changing her footwear (the probable cause of her pain) depends in part on her beliefs regarding the relation between fashion shoes and the development of her foot condition.
- **Severity** – This refers to the extent to which Suzi believes that hallux valgus is a serious condition.
- **Benefits and costs** – These factors combine to form Suzi's perception of the threat to her foot health and it is on this perception, together with the other factors shown in Figure 4.1, that Suzi will make a decision about changing her footwear. The model proposes that Suzi will weigh up the various benefits and costs of her taking any particular course of action (or of taking no action). From Suzi's perspective, the benefits of wearing fashionable shoes may outweigh the costs of developing hallux valgus.

Challenge 1: What are the bio-psychosocial risk factors for Suzi?

The first issue to consider is the ageing process. Bond & Coleman (1990) note that there is an inherent sexism attached to processes of ageing. While changes in physical appearance such as greying hair are seen as signs of increasing maturity in men, they are viewed as a waning of femininity in women. Suzi may be particularly vulnerable in this respect because of her occupation and the value that she attaches to her physical appearance.

A second important issue for Suzi is the prospect of the menopause, which usually commences in the fifth decade of life. Symptoms of the menopause include hot flushes and night sweats. It is also sometimes associated with low self-esteem, irritability and reduced libido. Other changes that occur at a similar time to the menopause may also impact on social identity and self-esteem. For example, children leaving home, divorce and elderly parents becoming dependent may result in considerable psychological upheaval.

Conversely, this period may be accompanied by a reappraisal of values and ambitions, which may result in greater contentment.

In addition to the psychological and physical changes that accompany the menopause, Suzi will have to consider the effects of osteoporosis. Osteoporosis is the commonest metabolic disease of bone and is most frequently found in women following the menopause. While the effects of osteoporosis are systemic, manifestations may also be found in the feet. Symptoms include pain, and sufferers are more susceptible to fractures. Smoking significantly increases the risk of developing osteoporosis.

On average, women who smoke reach the menopause up to 2 years earlier than women who are non-smokers. This is partly because chemicals in cigarette smoke reduce the levels of oestrogen in the blood. Smoking also constricts blood vessels, which leads to the exacerbation of symptoms such as hot flushes.

In Suzi's case, smoking and being menopausal combine in such a way that the sum is greater than a simple combination of the effects of these two factors. This effect is known as synergy.

The menopause is also a time that can be associated with an increase in weight. An increase in weight and change in body size and shape may have a negative effect on Suzi's self-image and self-esteem. In addition, it may increase the pain and discomfort she feels in her feet.

Self-esteem is concerned with how worthwhile and confident an individual feels about themselves. Self-esteem is a component of a complex self-system (Harter 1988a, b) which is composed of a number of components such as academic achievement, social acceptance, physical appearance and athletic ability. It may be viewed as either high or low depending on an individual's interpretation of their own abilities. It is also possible to have low scores for one component and still feel generally good about oneself. It is suggested that individuals have high self-esteem when the attributes that they like about themselves outweigh those that they dislike. This balance may be altered by life events (Fig. 4.2). In the case of significant events such as divorce, self-esteem may be decreased for extended periods of time (Harter 1985). In addition, transitional life stages may also exert a negative effect on self-esteem. Such episodes are described as 'mid-life crises' (Simmons et al 1983). The effect of conflict between an individual's notions about their ideal self and observations of their actual self may result in chronic anxiety or depression (Rogers 1951).

Suzi's self-esteem is likely to be affected by her recent divorce. Divorce is a common trigger for depression. Depression is characterized by sadness, low self-esteem, disturbed sleep patterns and weight gain or loss. Podiatrists need to be aware of the increasing divorce rate, which will inevitably bring them into contact with patients suffering the psychological effects of separation and divorce.

Finally, Suzi needs to consider that her footwear may be contributing to the painful and infected lesions between her toes that

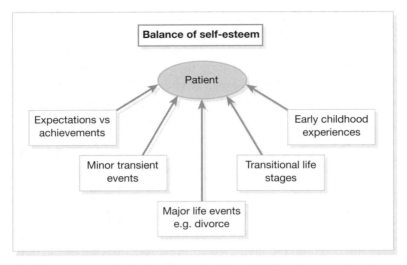

Fig. 4.2 Components of self-esteem (after Russell 1999, with permission of Routledge)

she presents with. One of the consequences of wearing inappropriate footwear may be a delay in the resolution of Suzi's infection.

Challenge 2: How might Suzi be helped?

You are concerned about the condition of Suzi's feet, and in particular the possible infection of her toes. For any of your treatment options to be successful, Suzi must begin to wear more sensible footwear. Therefore your first priority is to convince her of the benefits of such a change.

How to assist your patient to change

1. Identify the barriers to communication

In Suzi's case these barriers may consist of depression, stress, fear and anger. The podiatrist should listen, be empathetic and try to reach a point of common agreement. It is certainly essential to keep calm and avoid any confrontation. It is important to remain detached, making it clear that no personal criticism is implied in the conversation. Confrontation may lead to a heightened sense of arousal.

If Suzi indicates that she is considering making a formal complaint about the error in her appointment time, the podiatrist should always agree to investigate the substance of her complaint. It is also very important to be familiar with complaints procedure, should this become necessary. It is possible that an error in the appointment system has occurred, and the podiatrist must apologize if this is the case. If no error has occurred, then it is important to adopt an empathetic neutral approach.

Healthcare professionals also rely on non-verbal behaviour to aid communication. Empathy can be conveyed using appropriate non-verbal skills. Facial expression, eye contact, touch and proximity can help break down communication barriers. The use of appropriate volume, tone and pitch in speech can also defuse difficult communication situations effectively.

Suzi should be given the space and opportunity to articulate her problems and her perception of them. At the outset, Suzi may only talk about the superficial and immediate problems associated with her appointment. However, as trust becomes established, she may become more confident in the relationship and may be ready to discuss her more personal problems.

Once Suzi's agenda has been established, communication can progress. There may be occasions when the podiatrist and the patient have different expectations; the patient's expectations may be unrealistic. Conversely, the podiatrist may expect the patient to achieve more than is reasonable. It is therefore helpful during this phase to encourage the patient to discuss her treatment and prognosis expectations, and to negotiate realistic and achievable goals.

In the literature, communication is generally considered under the headings of verbal communication and non-verbal behaviour. Verbal communication is concerned with the spoken language. Language used when engaging in professional conversations should not be complicated by jargon and the delivery of information should be in manageable units that are understandable by the patient. Some useful techniques include phrases such as: 'What I am going to tell you now is important', or 'You need to listen carefully to what I am about to say', which alert the patient to the fact that what they are about to hear must be listened to and understood. Phrases such as this herald important information. Questioning styles may be open, allowing the respondent to elaborate their thoughts, feelings and concerns, much like the counselling style (McLoughlin 1996). Closed questions are best used to find out facts and only require simple yes/no responses. For example, a closed question might be: 'Is ibuprofen the only NSAID you take?' An open question on the same subject could be: 'What medication are you currently taking?' If a communication request is made, then even more information may be elicited, for example: 'Tell me about the medication you are currently taking'.

If the patient has difficulty understanding English, arrangements should be made for an interpreter to be present. The use of interpreters is discussed in Chapter 7.

Non-verbal behaviour is often called paralinguistics and is concerned with pace, tone, pitch, volume, dialect and pauses. It focuses on the way in which information is delivered, rather than what is actually said (Dickson et al 1997). Utterances may sometimes replace words, to provide feedback and regulate the speed at which a conversation progresses. Other components of non-verbal behaviour include touch, posture, position, gestures, facial expressions and personal proximity.

Touch is an important part of communication for the podiatrist. Professional touch is when the podiatrist touches the patient in order to carry out treatment, for example in the assessment of pulses and the range of joint motion and the reduction of corns and calluses. Therapeutic touch can be regarded as touch through which the therapeutic relationship is built, for example shaking hands or a sympathetic touch of the arm. It has been suggested that the position adopted by the podiatrist has a profound effect on the relationship that podiatrists develop with their patients (Mandy 2000).

Gesture and facial expression may be used to encourage or discourage engagement in communication. Eye contact is a technique that can be used to control communication and terminate it at an appropriate juncture (Dickson et al 1997).

Children are traditionally told to 'watch what they say'. Perhaps it would be better to tell them to 'watch what is said', as this would involve their learning to interpret the *meanings* of communication by reading non-verbal behaviour.

2. Identify the factors that will enable you to establish a therapeutic relationship

The podiatrist needs to make Suzi sufficiently comfortable within the relationship to discuss sensitive material that may affect her care. Frequently, patients are unaware of the impact that apparently unrelated factors can have on their foot health. For example, Suzi may not acknowledge that her menopause may be related to the development of hard skin on her heels and soles of her feet. Similarly, she may not associate the lesions on her toes with pressure and friction from footwear. In order to achieve a satisfactory relationship, the podiatrist should exhibit a warm, non-judgemental, open and caring approach. The podiatrist must actively *listen* to the patient.

As long ago as 1956, Szasz & Hollender described a model in which different typologies of relationships may be observed. 'Active/passive' typology is a term used to describe circumstances in which the therapist is the active participant, and the patient is solely a passive recipient of treatment. An example of this would be the comatose patient in the accident and emergency room who is attended to by the medical team. This typology is not usually encountered in podiatric practice.

In Szasz & Hollender's (1956) Guidance/Cooperative typology, it is assumed that the podiatrist has access to knowledge and information, which would therefore make the podiatrist equipped to offer advice and guidance, having taken the patient's wishes into account. In this typology, the podiatrist continues to dominate the question and answer sessions.

In the Mutual Participation typology, Szasz & Hollender (1956) propose that the consultation is characterized by a negotiation between both parties. The patient acknowledges the skill and expertise of the podiatrist, while retaining the right to decide on his/her own treatment.

In certain circumstances, Szasz & Hollender (1956) suggest a further typology, which they call Passive/Active. This situation exists when the patient is in possession of all the relevant facts concerning his/her condition, understands the treatment that is necessary and simply uses the podiatrist to provide it. Patients increasingly have access to relevant information using electronic sources such as the Internet, and are providing healthcare professionals with more challenging interactions (Neuberger 2000). Some practitioners may find this increased autonomy of patients difficult. Patient autonomy represents a shift of power within the relationship, with the potential for making the podiatrist feel that his/her position is being threatened.

The term 'concordance' is increasingly being used to describe the way in which a patient reacts to the advice and information offered by a practitioner. Many texts continue to use the terms 'adherence' and 'compliance' synonymously. The term concordance requires an understanding of the patient's health beliefs and an attempt to make them congruent with a course of action that will result in the maximum health gain. In Suzi's case, this will involve her choosing more appropriate footwear, using recommended medications and wearing appropriate orthotics.

Achieving concordance requires the podiatrist to be able to provide the necessary information in a way that is credible, understandable and acceptable to the patient. This may be achieved by developing communication skills and by the provision of written information that is presented in short sentences and uncomplicated language. The use of readability indices can help in ensuring that the message will be understood by potential readers. Readability indices are readily available on most personal computers.

In addition, when designing a treatment plan, patient and podiatrist should work together to provide an achievable regimen with realistic targets and time frames. Reinforcement should be built into the plan to assist in the achievement of targets and goals. When there is a complex regimen, it is often useful to suggest ways

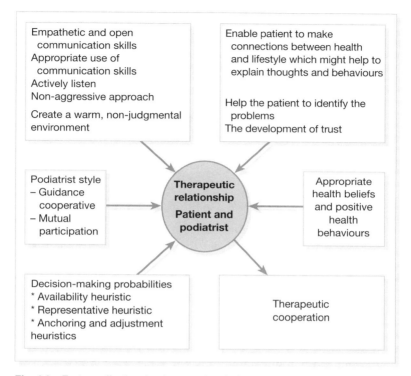

Fig. 4.3   Factors affecting the therapeutic relationship (Alder 1999)

in which tasks may be simplified. If patients can incorporate a task into their everyday life, it is more likely that they will undertake it: for example, encouraging a patient to apply foot cream after bathing will turn the task into a routine (Fig. 4.3).

Alder (1999) suggests that the process of making decisions does not always rely on logic but sometimes on perceived probabilities. The rules for working with probabilities are called heuristics, which can have potential biases (Alder 1999). These are defined as follows:

• The **availability heuristic** is a judgement based on available information about the subject of interest. Suzi may, for example, expect that her menopause is likely to occur during her 50s.

- The **representative heuristic** is a judgement based on information that is typical for a given group of people. Thus, if Suzi were to miss a period in her 50s, she might assume that she was menopausal, but during her 20s she might have suspected pregnancy.
- **Anchoring and adjustment heuristics** enable people to make judgements from a given starting point. For example, missing a period at the age of 47 might lead Suzi to think that she was experiencing her menopause earlier than her availability heuristic would suggest.

3. Achievement of therapeutic cooperation

It is necessary to understand why Suzi insists on wearing court shoes. Often, patients will insist that shoes that are potentially damaging to their feet are actually quite comfortable. The podiatrist will need to use skilled questioning in order to elicit when Suzi experiences pain and what she does to relieve her pain.

It is important that Suzi recognizes the role her shoes have in causing her symptoms and that she understands that other footwear may be more appropriate. It may be helpful to suggest that being more comfortable may influence her work performance positively and improve her general sense of wellbeing. At this point, Suzi may be more receptive to advice and more likely to consider a change in the style of her shoes. In addition, she will need information to help her to make informed choices.

If Suzi is unwilling to change her shoe style while at work, it may be possible to negotiate that she wears comfortable, well-fitting shoes during her leisure time. Such a compromise can often lead to full concordance with the treatment plan at a later date.

SUZI DALTON: SUMMARY OF IMPORTANT HEALTH PSYCHOLOGY

Communication is the key factor when treating patients such as Suzi. The use of appropriate communication skills enables the successful development of the therapeutic relationship. An understanding and application of the Health Belief Model will assist the podiatrist in helping Suzi change her foot-health behaviour. In addition, a better understanding of the more general psychological and physiological factors influencing Suzi's current behaviour is valuable in this process.

In particular, podiatrists should be aware of the impact that menopausal symptoms can have on their patients' physical and psychological wellbeing.

FURTHER READING

Boyd D, Stevens G 2001 Current readings in life span development. Allyn & Bacon, Boston, MA

Dickson DA, Hargie O, Morrow NC 1997 Communication skills training for health professionals: an instructor's handbook. Chapman & Hall, London

REFERENCES

Alder B 1999 Psychology of health: applications of health psychology for health professionals, 2nd edn. Harwood Academic Publishers, New York

Becker MH, Rosenstock IM 1984 Compliance with medical advice. In Steptoe A, Mathews A (ed) Healthcare and human behaviour. Academic Press, London

Bond J, Coleman P 1990 (ed) Ageing in society: an introduction to social gerontology. Sage, London

Dickson DA, Hargie O, Morrow NC 1997 Communication skills training for health professionals: an instructor's handbook, 2nd edn. Chapman & Hall, London

Harter S 1985 Competence as a dimension of self-evaluation. Towards a comprehensive model of self worth. In Leahy RL (ed) The development of the self. Academic Press, Orlando, FL

Harter S 1988a The determinations and mediations of global self-worth in children. In Eisberg N (ed) Contemporary topics in developmental psychology. Wiley-Interscience, New York

Harter S 1988b Developmental processes in the construction of the self. In Yankey TD, Johnson JE (ed) Integrative processes and socialism: early to middle childhood. John Wiley, New York

McLoughlin B 1996 Developing psychodynamic counselling, 2nd edn. Sage, London

Mandy P 2000 The nature and status of chiropody and dentistry. DPhil thesis, University of Sussex

Neuberger 2000 The educated patient: new challenges for the medical profession. Journal of Internal Medicine 247, 6–10

Rogers C 1951 Client centred therapy. Houghton Mifflin, Boston, MA

Russell G 1999 Essential psychology. Routledge, London

Simmons RG, Blyth DA, McKinney KL 1983 The social and psychological effects of puberty on white females. In Brooks-Gunn J, Petersen AC (ed) Girls and puberty: biological and psychological perspectives. Plenum Press, New York

Szasz TS, Hollender MH 1956 A contribution to the philosophy of medicine: the basic models of the doctor–patient relationship. Archives of Internal Medicine 97, 585–592

5

Charles Walters – problems of retirement and the sickness role

We are responsible for actions performed in response to
circumstances for which we are not responsible.

Allan Massie

Charles is a 52-year-old ex-policeman who has been retired early
on medical grounds. In the past 5 years, he has developed
maturity-onset diabetes, which he has been unable to control by
modification of his diet, and therefore has to take tablets. He is
overweight and does not take any exercise. Charles had worked
for the police force since leaving school at 16 years of age. He was
committed to his chosen career and it fulfilled his life. He is not
married and, because of his lifelong commitment to his work, has
found the transition into early retirement difficult. He has few
interests outside work and has not had time to develop any social
activities. He recognizes that his diabetes has got worse and
admits that he finds it difficult to control his diet and thinks he is
too old to take up any sport.

Charles knows that he is eligible for podiatry treatment because
of his diabetes.

Charles presents with only minor podiatric problems but he
attends the podiatry clinic regularly for assessment and monitoring. As part of the multiprofessional team who are involved in
diabetic care, the podiatrist will not only assess his neurological
and vascular status but will also be concerned with preventing
the development of diabetic complications.

FACTORS THAT INFLUENCE CHARLES'S BEHAVIOUR

Charles has good intentions regarding his diabetes but, in his own words, he 'enjoys his food'. However, he also believes that the services provided by the 'specialist' healthcare workers will be more influential in controlling his diabetes than any actions of his own, because 'they are the professionals'. As a result, he has become quite dependent on all the people in the clinics he attends. Charles's diet is not very well controlled, and it is important that the podiatrist understands how Charles makes choices about what he eats.

A number of theories have been proposed that try to explain how people make health-related decisions. These models are known collectively as social cognition models, and many applications are noted in the health psychology literature. One of the most important of these is the theory of reasoned action (Fishbein & Ajzen 1975; Fig. 5.1).

In this case, Charles's behavioural beliefs may include:

- Eating a healthy diet will help reduce the complications of my diabetes
- Eating a healthy diet will help me lose weight
- Eating a healthy diet will improve my ability to heal.

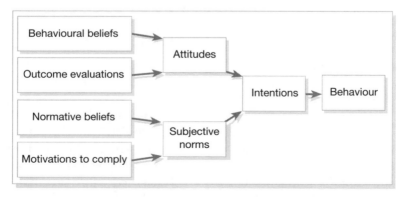

Fig. 5.1 The theory of reasoned action (Fishbein & Ajzen 1975, after Sutton 1989. © John Wiley & Sons Limited. Reproduced with permission.)

All the outcome evaluations corresponding to these beliefs are likely to be positive.

Conversely, Charles's behavioural beliefs may also include:

- A healthy diet is boring
- Being unable to drink with my friends restricts my social life
- I'd have to give up all the things I like if I ate a healthy diet.

All the outcome evaluations corresponding to these beliefs are likely to be negative.

These conflicting behavioural beliefs and evaluations combine to produce Charles's attitudes to changing his diet.

Charles's normative beliefs concerning eating a healthy diet may include:

- My specialists think that improving my diet would help my diabetes
- The people managing my treatment are experts in diabetes.

Charles's motivations to comply may include:

- I want to please the specialists who are looking after me
- Experts know best, so I'll try really hard to diet.

However, Charles's normative beliefs concerning eating a healthy diet may also include:

- Being among my old workmates is more important than what doctors tell you.

And his motivations to comply may include:

- I'm not going to be told what to do by so-called experts.

These conflicting normative beliefs and motivations combine to produce Charles's subjective norms in relation to changing his diet. Charles's behavioural beliefs and subjective norms in turn combine to influence his intention to either change his diet or continue his previous pattern of eating.

If the podiatrist can influence Charles's beliefs and thus his attitudes toward changing his diet, this may increase the likelihood of changing his intentions in that area. Such influence is very dependent on the quality of the therapeutic relationship that is

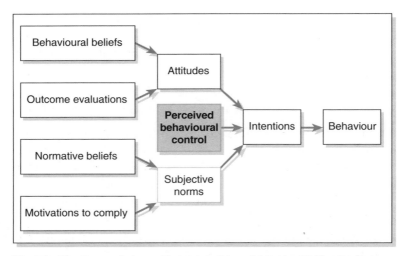

Fig. 5.2 The theory of planned behaviour (Ajzen & Madden 1986, after Sutton 1989. © John Wiley & Sons Limited. Reproduced with permission.)

formed between the podiatrist, Charles and the diabetic team. The nature and importance of the therapeutic relationship is described in Chapter 4.

A variant of the theory of reasoned action that has attracted considerable attention recently is the theory of planned behaviour (Ajzen & Madden 1986; Fig. 5.2). In addition to the components of the theory of reasoned action, a further element is included, which is known as perceived behavioural control. This component is a direct measure of the degree of control that the individual feels s/he has over the behaviour in question. Perceived behavioural control is an important addition to the model, particularly in the case of behaviours with an addictive component, for example smoking, drinking or other drug use.

For many years, the theory of planned behaviour has been used in attempts to explain a wide range of health-related behaviours. Applications include studies of cigarette smoking, alcohol and drug use, exercise behaviour, concordance with medical treatments and dietary advice. However, the models such as the theory of reasoned action and theory of planned behaviour have a number of shortcomings, which have recently become widely recognized among health psychologists (e.g. Roberts et al 2001). Notably, the models assume that people act in a logical and rational way that many consider to be unrealistic. Secondly, while subjective norms and attitudes predict intentions quite well in statistical analyses, the models' overall ability to predict actual behaviour is limited. Perhaps most importantly, such models fail to appreciate the complexity of the social context in which most health-related behaviours are located.

The sick role was a concept introduced by Parsons in 1951. Parsons defined health as a 'state of optimum capacity for effective role performance'. Conversely, illness is a generalized disturbance of this state. Where role capacity is affected by illness the individual is given a status and role in society, that of the 'sick' person. The sick role is characterized by rights and obligations for both the sick person and the practitioner. There are four main features of the sick role:

• The sick person is exempted from the performance of his/her social duties. This exemption requires validation by others, especially medical practitioners, who have been given the power to determine whether a person is sick or not.

• The sick person is not held responsible for his/her state of health. Therefore the sick person cannot be asked to 'pull yourself together and get better'.

• The sick person is obliged to give up the right to engage in activities normally undertaken by healthy people. If a person suffering from a heavy cold has adopted the sick role and taken a day off from work s/he is not then entitled, according to the sick role, to go out the same evening to engage in a social event.

• The sick person is obliged to seek qualified help where appropriate and to follow the advice of a qualified practitioner.

Charles is happy to accept some of the rights of the sick role but few of the obligations.

The term 'diabetes mellitus' describes a metabolic disorder of multiple aetiology characterized by chronic hyperglycaemia with disturbances of carbohydrate, fat and protein metabolism resulting from defects in insulin secretion, insulin action or both (World

Health Organization 1999). The effects of diabetes mellitus include long-term damage, dysfunction and failure of various organs.

The long-term effects of diabetes mellitus include progressive development of the specific complications of retinopathy with potential blindness, nephropathy, which may lead to renal failure, and/or neuropathy with risk of foot ulcers, amputation, Charcot's joints and features of autonomic dysfunction, including sexual dysfunction. People with diabetes are at increased risk of cardio-vascular, peripheral vascular and cerebrovascular disease.

Diabetes mellitus can be classified into two types. The majority of Type I cases are primarily due to pancreatic islet beta-cell destruction and are prone to ketoacidosis. Type I includes those cases attributable to an autoimmune process, as well as those with beta-cell destruction and those who are prone to ketoacido-sis for which neither an aetiology nor a pathogenesis is known (idiopathic).

Type II diabetes includes the common major form of diabetes, which results from a defect(s) in insulin secretion, almost always with a major contribution from insulin resistance.

Diabetes is a common metabolic disorder, which attracts many misconceptions regarding its course and treatment. There is strong convincing evidence to show that good control of blood sugar reduces the development of the common diabetic complica-tions, including nephropathy, neuropathy, retinopathy and vas-cular disease. It is now accepted that good diabetic control is achieved by following a healthy, balanced diet, taking regular exercise, avoiding too much alcohol and stopping smoking. This advice is common for the entire population and not directed at those people with diabetes.

Challenge 1: Identify why you think it is difficult for Charles to follow a healthy lifestyle

Charles has a history of eating institutional food, which tradition-ally has a high fat content and low nutritional value. He is also used to having his food prepared for him and is not experienced in either shopping for or preparing food. He continues to enjoy canteen food and is therefore reluctant to learn how to prepare and cook food for himself. He considers what most nutritionists regard as healthy food to be effete.

Charles also believes that he is physically fit, having spent years 'walking the beat' as a policeman, and is reluctant to engage in any organized forms of exercise. He believes it to be unnecessary for him. Charles is used to his lifestyle and any suggestions regarding changes in his behaviour tend to make him feel challenged and uncomfortable.

Consider what other factors may be important in influencing Charles's behaviour that are not included within the theory of reasoned action and theory of planned behaviour.

Challenge 2: What strategies could you employ to persuade Charles to review his current behaviour?

The terms 'multiprofessional', 'interdisciplinary' and 'multidisciplinary' are often used synonymously. The multiprofessional team consists of a range of different healthcare professionals, and also social-care professionals, who work together for the benefit of the patient. The core team involved with Charles's care may include a diabetic consultant, a diabetic nurse specialist, a dietitian and podiatrists, who would meet to assess and review the provision of care and advice being provided. Others, for instance a clinical psychologist, prosthetist, microbiologist, etc., are included as required. Each member of the team will contribute a specialist understanding of their role and will develop an understanding of each other's roles. They will also contribute team-working skills and positive attitudes, which afford successful interprofessional interaction.

Successful multiprofessional teamwork learning involves the development of shared strategies for clinical and professional interventions.

The team involved in the diabetic care of Charles are all actively involved in providing support and reinforcing appropriate behaviours. In order for Charles to achieve his goals, he needs to be provided with information delivered in such a way that he can see the personal benefits of changing his behaviours without compromising his lifestyle. His treatment plan should be designed in such a way as to offer Charles small achievable targets towards the achievement of the overall goal. Positive reinforcement is essential at each stage of the treatment plan and this should be carefully determined and agreed with Charles. All messages should be kept short. When written information is given to Charles, it should be presented in a comprehensible form. Changes to Charles's lifestyle are more likely to occur if they can be integrated into his daily routine.

To improve Charles's health, he does not need to give up his visits to the police social club but simply to choose healthier options on the menu and moderate his alcohol intake. In addition, he would be helped by taking up a hobby or pastime that involves an element of physical exercise, such as walking or cycling. Charles may wish to begin by walking at least some of the way to and from his club.

Self-help groups such as Diabetes UK offer a useful service to people who are newly diagnosed as having diabetes. Such groups offer support, information, guidance and friendship from other people with diabetes. Increasingly, patients are using recommended web pages from the Internet to gather information about their condition. The Internet also offers the opportunity to exchange views, information and opinions.

There is also an important issue concerning being prepared for retirement and consideration of life after work. For people who have not prepared adequately, retirement can be a stressful event. Giving up work can be perceived as losing something that is very important. Most employees spend a great deal of time at work, invest effort, energy and enthusiasm, and in return gain satisfaction and a sense of belonging and self-worth. When retirement is not planned, or is enforced, feelings of loss may trigger physical and emotional reactions.

People previously in senior positions may suffer from the associated loss of status and may resent the loss of seniority that may have taken years to acquire. In all cases, retirement is associated with a loss of income. There may also be feelings of loss of purpose and structure to the day. Employment involves decision making, interaction with other employees, the experience of the highs and lows of work life and the physical effort of being at work for designated periods of time. Employees are often known for their role in the workplace, and thus retirement may result in the loss of social identity.

While many people look forward to retirement, it can also be a source of great stress. Many organizations now offer preretirement courses to help prepare their employees to make the transition from work to retirement successful.

CHARLES WALTERS: SUMMARY OF IMPORTANT HEALTH PSYCHOLOGY

Social–psychological models that try to explain behaviour in general may be helpful when considering an individual patient, but advice should be given in the context of the patient's own individual circumstances.

It is important for Charles to address the issues of retirement and develop interests and activities that will result in him being able to lead a fulfilled and healthier life.

FURTHER READING

Anon 1999 The psychology of retirement: how to cope successfully with a major life transition. By The Everyday Psychologist. Business Psychology Research Institute, Arlington Heights, IL

Eysenck MW 2000 Psychology: a students handbook. Psychology Press, Brighton

Naidoo J, Wills J 1994 Health promotion: foundations for practice. Baillière Tindall, London

Roberts R, Golding JF, Towell T 2001 Foundations of health psychology. Palgrave, Basingstoke

---

REFERENCES

Ajzen I, Madden TJ 1986 Prediction of goal-directed behavior: attitudes intentions, and perceived behavioral control. Journal of Experimental Social Psychology 22, 453–474

Fishbein M, Ajzen I 1975 Belief, attitudes, intentions and behaviour: an introduction to theory. Addison-Wesley, New York

Parsons T 1951 The social system. Free Press, Glencoe, IL

Roberts R, Golding JF, Towell T 2001 Foundations of health psychology. Palgrave, Basingstoke

Sutton SR 1989 Smoking attitudes and behaviours: applications of Fishbein and Ajzen's theory of reasoned action to predicting and understanding smoking decisions. In Ney T, Gale A (eds) Smoking and human behaviour. John Wiley & Sons, Chichester

World Health Organization 1999 Definition, diagnosis and classification of diabetes mellitus and its complications. WHO, Geneva

6

James Watt – problems of personality and addictive behaviour

The tragedy of machismo is that a man is never quite man enough.

Germaine Greer

James Watt is a 31-year-old runner who has been referred for the first time to the podiatrist. The podiatrist is Jenny, the young and recently qualified graduate introduced in Chapter 2. James is employed as a sales executive for a local insurance company, which he joined straight from school. He has progressed rapidly through the company and feels that he has been successful as a result of hard work. He questions the need for 'university education' as a key to success and believes that 'everyone could be successful if they worked hard enough'. The major part of James's income is derived from commission. He likes this arrangement as he is ambitious, competitive and approaches his work aggressively. James is generally sociable, enjoys bars, pubs and clubs and has a wide circle of friends and associates from his work. He uses the gym two or three times a week but his major leisure activity is running. James considers himself to be a competitive runner and is a member of the local harriers. He runs, on average, about 30 miles a week. James believes that running keeps him 'sharp' and gives him an 'edge' in both his social and work life. He enjoys female company but finds it difficult to maintain relationships because of his condescending attitude towards women.

James presents with pain in the anterior aspect of the lower limb, which he describes as 'shin splints'. This condition is considered to be an overuse syndrome.

FACTORS THAT INFLUENCE JAMES'S BEHAVIOUR

James works in an environment that he finds stimulating and satisfying but that is competitive and financially driven. Being fit is extremely important to him because he believes fitness helps him to work more effectively and he also likes the 'buzz' that competitive running provides. His body image is very important to him and he feels confident that he has up-to-date knowledge about how to maintain his physique. He presents with a distinct air of arrogance and is patronizing in his manner.

IMPORTANT PSYCHOLOGICAL THEORY

Theories of social perception help to describe how instant assessments of patients occur. Early work by Asch (1946) suggested that impressions are drawn from general characteristics and that individuals draw upon their own social constructions of beliefs about people. First impressions can be an important influence, and physical attractiveness has also been shown to be an significant factor. The more physically attractive an individual is deemed to be, the more likely they are to be perceived as intelligent, competent and sociable. For podiatrists, it is important not to make such judgements.

Personality is considered to be sufficiently stable over time for it to be assessed in order to predict behaviour. Many writers have proposed models of personality, which have attracted proponents and antagonists in equal measure.

Friedman & Rosenman (1974) identified two basic personality types, which they used to describe differences in behaviour. They labelled individuals as either type A or type B depending on whether they displayed certain characteristics and behavioural responses. Type A individuals tend to be competitive, achievement-orientated and impatient, hostile and aggressive and have a sense of urgency about tasks. Conversely, Type B individuals are characterized by non-competitiveness, patience and a placid temperament. Although there has been much research into the relationship between type A personality and disease, in particular coronary heart disease, there is little corresponding work focusing on the effects of a type B personality. More recently, a further personality type (labelled C) has been posited, which is characterized by a habitual tendency to suppress emotions. This tendency has been associated with a number of negative health outcomes. For example, in two longitudinal studies Grosarth-Maticek et al (1982) found emotional suppression to be a significant predictor of cancer in women.

However, there is now wide acceptance of the personality structure proposed by McCrae & Costa (1987). They describe five 'factors' that define an individual's personality. This model has come to be known widely as the Five Factor Theory or 'Big Five' model. The five factors are:

- **Openness to experience**: the extent to which an individual is willing to try new things
- **Conscientiousness**: the extent to which the individual tends to be committed to tasks
- **Extroversion**: the extent to which the individual is outgoing
- **Agreeableness**: the extent to which the individual gets on well with others
- **Neuroticism**: individuals scoring highly tend to feel insecure and to worry.

The structure proposed by the 'Big Five' model has been supported by much statistical evidence. It may be remembered easily by the use of the mnemonic OCEAN.

Personality is believed to influence behaviour profoundly. People who score at the extremes, either high or low, on any of the factors described above are likely to present challenges when attempting to alter their behaviour. This will be the case when Jenny works with James Watt.

Challenge 1: Identify the psychological factors that need to be taken into account when planning a treatment regime for James

Jenny must help James to appreciate the importance of modifying his training regime in order to achieve full rehabilitation and enable him to return to competitive running. In order to be able to do this effectively, she will need to understand that running competitively is in part a product of his personality. In addition, running provides James with the opportunity to maintain his appearance, which he values highly.

The 'runner's high' is a recognized state found in long-distance runners. Endorphins are neurotransmitters that are chemically similar to morphine and are thought to be responsible for elevating mood and reducing pain, particularly after intense periods of exercise such as running. Running has also been associated with feelings of invincibility and superiority (Weston 1996). The physiological 'high' produced by endorphins in runners is an additional reinforcer of James's running behaviour.

It is necessary, therefore, to identify an alternative means of meeting these needs on a temporary basis while James stops running in order for resolution of his condition to take place. Although the initial need for rest is of paramount importance, replacement activities must also be considered, discussed and negotiated.

James's personality is such that he is likely to demand simple answers to solve his problem, thereby enabling him to carry on his fitness regime. Jenny will be helped in this task by an understanding of personality theory and how personality may influence health-related behaviour. Jenny's approach should thus be a combination of empathy and assertiveness.

Jenny's task is complicated further by the interaction of James's personality and the pain he experiences. Pain is a common experience and is inseparable from everyday life. Physiologically, pain can be considered as an unpleasant sensory and emotional experience associated with actual or potential tissue damage. The physiological process of pain is described extensively in appropriate texts and is not the focus of this book. Understanding psychological responses to pain is very important for podiatrists. The way in which an individual responds to pain will vary according to certain factors, which are outlined below.

Factors affecting pain perception

The following factors all impact on the experience and expression of pain:

- Social and cultural background
- Previous experiences of pain
- The responses of significant others to pain
- Emotional effects
- The perceived intensity of the pain
- The ability to communicate and describe the pain
- Permission to express pain in the culture
- The efficacy of pain-relieving drugs.

Interprofessional communication

It is important to establish James's source of referral and his treatment history. If he has sought the advice of several other professionals prior to being referred to the podiatrist, it is important that Jenny obtains this information early on and determines the nature of the advice he has been given. If the advice Jenny provides is congruent with advice James has been given earlier, then he is more likely to follow it.

Jenny's communication style needs to be confident, knowledgeable and sensitive to James's needs. She should be aware of, and understand, the factors that make running so important to James.

It is also necessary for James to listen actively to the advice Jenny gives in order that an agreed treatment plan can be devised.

Challenge 2: Identify the potential problems you might encounter with James and how you would overcome them

Addictive behaviours

'Addiction' is a term that is often used somewhat loosely, and some authors have pointed out that it is not only substances such as alcohol, nicotine and opiates that have 'addictive' properties. Many of the features of such substances can also be seen in certain behaviours, notably in the case of athletic and sporting endeavour. In a slightly whimsical overview of the debate, Miller & Marlatt

(1977) describe a screening test for an addictive state they describe as 'skiism'. They observe that skiing is 'a winter sport/addictive behaviour of major proportions' and note that its victims persist with their addiction 'in spite of the ever-increasing cost of their habit, and seemingly oblivious to the steady stream of ambulances that carry off the casualties of intemperance and over-exposure'. Miller & Marlatt (1977) propose a psychological self-assessment scale, which suggests that positive responses to such questions as 'Has skiing ever separated you from your family?' and 'Do you find that it takes progressively stiffer slopes to satisfy you?' indicate a condition that Stepney (1981) describes as 'the features of escapism, development of tolerance, and personal and social dislocation which characterize a full-blown dependence disorder'. Symptoms of exercise addiction can also include non-compliance, aggression and the need to continually seek advice from different healthcare professionals.

Viewed from this perspective, the notion of a 'jogging addiction' seems less absurd than a first glance might suggest. James exhibits many features of addictive behaviour and it is important that Jenny gives them adequate consideration in agreeing the treatment plan.

Aggression

Aggression may manifest in many forms, the nature of which may be mediated by factors such gender, age and culture. Aggression may be considered as behaviour or speech intended to harm someone else, to obtain material goods or as a reaction to another person's aggressive behaviour.

Research indicates that men have a tendency to be more aggressive than women, largely because of their different characteristic levels of the hormone testosterone. However, Bjorkqvist et al (1992) studied physical, verbal and indirect aggression (such as gossiping and writing unkind notes) in adolescent males and females. They found that boys displayed higher levels of physical aggression but girls showed significantly higher level of indirect aggression. Boys and girls showed no difference in their levels of verbal aggression.

One of the most influential approaches to understanding aggression is social learning theory, first proposed by Bandura (1973). This theory suggests that aggressive behaviour is the product of 'observational learning' or copying the behaviour of others. Bandura's theory is limited in that it does not take into account factors such as a person's affective state, their interpretation of their situation or their personality. A more recent theory of aggression has been proposed by proponents of social constructionism. Social constructionists such as Gergen (1997) believe that people impose subjective interpretations or constructions on the environment surrounding them. When applied to aggression, social constructionism is based on the following assumptions:

- Aggressive behaviour is a form of social behaviour and is not simply the expression of anger
- Our interpretation or construction of someone else's behaviour as aggressive or non-aggressive depends on our beliefs and knowledge
- Our decision whether to behave aggressively or non-aggressively depends on how we interpret the other person's behaviour to us (Gergen 1997).

The value of this approach is that it takes into consideration the effect of attitudes and beliefs and the need to distinguish between what actually happens in a social situation and what is perceived to happen. Conversely, a criticism that could be applied is that social constructionist approaches may exaggerate the differences between different individuals' constructions of what has occurred.

All healthcare practitioners have an important role to play in helping achieve concordance with negotiated treatment plans. Providing patients with clear, honest explanations and advice, while being sensitive to their individual needs, promotes concordance (Pitts 1991). Other strategies include keeping a diary, graduating the complexity of the prescribed regimen, marrying the requirements of the regimen to daily activities and finding alternatives for the behaviour that the patient finds difficult to change. For example, James could use weights or swim in order to maintain his fitness during the necessary period of rest.

JAMES WATT: SUMMARY OF IMPORTANT HEALTH PSYCHOLOGY

The important psychological issues in this case study surround the manifestations of James's personality in his behaviour. James obtains satisfaction from the challenges that he has built into his life, which include working on a commission basis and the competitive nature of his relaxation activities. An understanding of his nature and motivations will enable Jenny to build a rehabilitation programme with which James is likely to be concordant. In addition, she must understand and acknowledge that patients interpret pain differently and also respond in individual ways to pain.

FURTHER READING

Adams L, Amos M, Munro J 2002 Promoting health. Sage, London
Eysenck, MW 2000 Psychology: a students handbook, 4th edn. Psychology Press, Brighton
Higdon H 1998 Hal Higdon's smart running : expert advice on training, motivation, injury prevention, nutrition, and good health for runners of any age and ability. Rodale Press, Emmaus, PA
Skevington, SM 1995 Psychology of pain. John Wiley, New York

REFERENCES

Asch SE 1946 Forming impressions of personality. Journal of Abnormal and Social Psychology 41, 258–290
Bandura A 1973 Aggression: a social learning analysis. Prentice Hall, Englewood Cliffs, NJ
Bjorkqvist K, Lagerspetz KMJ, Kaukiainen A 1992 Do girls manipulate and boys fight? Developmental trends regarding direct and indirect aggression. Aggressive Behaviour 18, 157–166
Friedman M, Rosenman RH 1974 Type A behaviour and your heart. Knopf, New York
Gergen KJ 1997 Social psychology as social construction: the emerging vision. In McGarty C, Haslam A (ed) The message of social psychology. Blackwell, Oxford
Grosarth-Maticek R, Kanariz DT, Schmidt P 1982 Psychosomatic processes in the development of cancerogenesis. Psychotherapy and Psychosomatics 38, 284–302
McCrae RR, Costa PJ Jr 1987 Validation of the five factor model of personality across instruments and observers. Journal of Personality and Social Psychology 52, 81–90

Miller WR, Marlatt, GA 1977 The Banff Skiism Test: an instrument for assessing degree of addiction. Addictive Behaviours 11, 49–53

Pitts M 1991 The experience of treatment. In Pitts M, Phillips K (eds) The psychology of health. Routledge, London

Stepney R 1981 Habits and addictions. Bulletin of the British Psychological Society 34, 233–235

Weston Drew 1996 Psychology: mind brain & culture. John Wiley & Son, New York

7

Sheetal Joshi – a patient from an ethnic minority

Shallow understanding from people of good will is more frustrating than absolute misunderstanding from people of ill will.

Martin Luther King Jr

Sheetal is a 70-year-old Asian woman, born in the Indian subcontinent, who does not speak any English. She is dressed in a traditional style of clothing that covers her head, arms and legs. Sheetal is small, slightly overweight, grey-haired and had a stroke about a year ago that affected the right side of her body. Her arm is fixed in a flexed position, her gait is affected and she has to walk with the aid of a walking stick.

Sheetal lives with her extended family in a predominantly Asian community in London. She is a devout Muslim. She is accompanied by her daughter-in-law, Hetal, who speaks good English and, since Sheetal was widowed, has acted as her interpreter. Sheetal both communicates through Hetal and consults her when asked questions. She does not maintain eye contact with anyone other than her daughter-in-law, and looks to her for confirmation that her responses are 'correct'. Sheetal believes that her stroke and resultant disability are 'God's way of testing her faith'.

Hetal reports that, since having had her stroke, her mother-in-law has become depressed and that she is reluctant to go out of the house. Sheetal is afraid of falling and feels that if she were to have an accident she would not be able to make herself understood in order to get help. Hetal also reports that her mother-in-law feels frustrated by her lack of improvement over the last few months.

Sheetal has been referred to the podiatrist for an assessment of her foot health and rehabilitation options. Her doctor is concerned about her vascular status and the care of her feet. He has referred her for advice and treatment, which may include orthotic management.

FACTORS THAT INFLUENCE SHEETAL'S BEHAVIOUR

Asian people living in the UK have been found to have high rates of stroke, which are attributed to high dietary salt and sugar intake (Enas et al 1996, 1997). Stroke is the leading form of cardiovascular disease in Asian populations (Enas et al 1997).

A stroke is a disruption in the blood supply to the brain. It is frequently referred to as a cerebrovascular accident, or CVA for short. It is also discussed in terms of left CVA or right CVA, referring to the left or right hemisphere of the brain. If the disruption is temporary and blood flow is restored without any residual or remaining difficulty, then the episode is known as a transient ischaemic attack (TIA). If the disruption in blood supply is not restored, permanent damage to the affected brain tissue will ensue, which leads to the muscular dysfunctions and deformities associated with stroke.

Asian immigrants to the UK are known to use health services less often and suffer more from premature death, disease and disabilities than do people born in the UK. Many also face social, economic and cultural barriers to maintaining good health. Because ethnic minority groups in the UK are very diverse, women's access to healthcare, their health behaviours and their health status can vary widely. Depression is a commonly reported psychological outcome of stroke.

This is the first time the podiatrist has met Sheetal and her daughter-in-law. The letter of referral provides limited information and only a sketchy medical history. It is important for the podiatrist to have an understanding of the relevant cultural issues in order to be able to provide Sheetal with appropriate podiatric care and advice.

IMPORTANT PSYCHOSOCIAL FACTORS

Sheetal's religious and cultural background would make her very unwilling to expose any part of her body to a male podiatrist. She may ask if there is a female podiatrist available but this should be anticipated and provided without the need for her to make such a request. Sheetal's attitudes towards her health will be closely interwoven with her religious beliefs.

South Asians living in the UK (Indians, Bangladeshis, Pakistanis and Sri Lankans), have a higher than average premature death rate from coronary heart disease. The rate is 46% higher for men and 51% higher for women.

The difference in the death rates between South Asians and the rest of the British population is increasing as the mortality rate in Asian people is not falling as fast as it is in the rest of the population. From 1971–91 the mortality rate in 20–69-year-olds for the whole population fell by 29% for men and 17% for women. In South Asian people it fell by 20% for men and 7% for women. South Asian people also have a mortality rate from stroke that is 55% higher than average for men and 41% higher for women.

The association between depression and stroke is well established in terms of its negative impact on an individual's rehabilitation, family relationships, and their subsequent quality of life. The early diagnosis and treatment of depression can shorten the rehabilitation period, and lead to more rapid recovery and resumption of routine daily activities.

Conducting an interview through an interpreter will require more time than would a similar interaction with an English-speaking patient. This should be borne in mind when allocating appointment times. Some of the finer points of the conversation may be lost in interpretation. Moreover, people from different cultures may use non-verbal signals in ways that may be unfamiliar or open to misinterpretation. Interpreters have the responsibility of passing on complex information or material that is personal or sensitive in nature, and about which the patient may have to make decisions.

The use of an interpreter may result in the patient feeling embarrassed or intimidated, particularly if the interpreter is from a higher social class or, as in Sheetal's case, a family member. If the interpreter is from the same community as the patient there may be anxieties concerning the disclosure of intimate family matters and associated issues of confidentiality (Karseras & Hopkins 1987). In addition, Hetal may feel embarrassed by her mother-in-law's inability to speak English and her possible lack of understanding of her condition and may wish to compensate by implying that Sheetal understands things when in reality she may not.

Traditionally, on marriage, the bride and her new husband live with her in-laws and she regards her mother-in-law as a mentor who will provide guidance and advice. Mothers and wives have clearly defined roles within the family unit. However, during Sheetal's visit to the clinic, these roles are reversed. Sheetal is completely dependent upon Hetal's ability to speak English and is thus disempowered. By contrast, Hetal may feel apprehensive about accepting this atypical role, with the responsibility of ensuring satisfactory provision of her mother-in-law's healthcare.

Challenge 1: How can you be sure that the patient's needs are being presented accurately? How can you feel confident that the information and advice offered is understood?

The tripartite nature of the consultation (Fig. 7.1) may lead to Hetal translating verbatim, interpreting the messages and responses, or a mixture of these. This may lead to inaccuracies in the understandings between Sheetal and the podiatrist, which may result in inappropriate treatment and advice.

In the process of interpretation many subtleties of conversation may be lost. The relative emphasis placed on different components in the exchange, for example history-taking, severity and duration of symptoms (from Sheetal via Hetal to the podiatrist) and information, advice and education (from the podiatrist to Sheetal via Hetal) may be altered. This may result in a compromised outcome for both patient and podiatrist. A useful technique that may be helpful in this situation is to invite the interpreter to paraphrase your original message from time to time during the consultation.

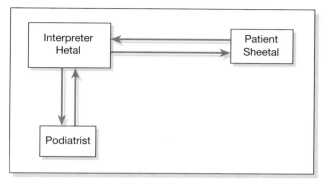

Fig. 7.1 Communication and the interpreter – note that there is no direct communication between the podiatrist and Sheetal: all the communication occurs through Hetal

Challenge 2: Consider the central role of religious beliefs in people's lives

Many studies have demonstrated the positive effects of religiosity on a wide range of health outcomes, for example reductions in coronary heart disease (Koenig et al 1998), hypertension and cancer (Levin 1994). It is therefore important to understand religion or spirituality as a central feature of many people's lives, rather than as a potential barrier to treatment (Koenig 1998).

SHEETAL JOSHI: SUMMARY OF IMPORTANT PSYCHOLOGICAL FACTORS

The podiatrist will require sensitivity and patience in order to meet Sheetal's needs. Sheetal's inability to speak English and the residual effects of her recent stroke will make communication difficult. In addition, cultural and religious understanding is essential to Sheetal's successful rehabilitation.

FURTHER READING

Helman C 2000 Culture, health and illness, 4th edn. Butterworth-Heinemann, Oxford

Morris DB 1998 Illness and culture in the postmodern age. University of California Press, Berkeley, CA
Lupton D 1994 Medicine as culture: illness, disease and the body in western societies. Sage, London

REFERENCES

Enas EA, Dhawan J, Petkar S 1997 Coronary artery disease in Asian Indians: lessons learnt and the role of lipoprotein. Indian Heart Journal 49, 25–34
Enas EA, Yusuf S, Mehta J 1996 Coronary artery disease in South Asians. Meeting of the International Working Group. Indian Heart Journal 48, 727–732
Karseras P, Hopkins E 1987 British Asians. Health in the community. John Wiley, Chichester
Koenig HG 1998 Religious attitudes and practices of hospitalized medically ill older adults. International Journal of Geriatric Psychiatry 13, 213–224
Koenig HG, George LK, Hays JC et al 1998 The relationship between religious activities and blood pressure in older adults. International Journal of Psychiatry in Medicine 28, 189–213
Levin JS 1994 Religion and health: is there an association, is it valid and is it causal? Social Science and Medicine 38, 1475–1482

8

Enid Hilton – a recently bereaved elderly lady

*If two people love each other there can be no happy
end to it.*

Ernest Hemingway

Enid Hilton moved from the Midlands to retire to the south coast with her husband. She has been living in the town with her husband in a small flat for 10 years. She is a smart, slender lady who always seems to wear a hat and coat and low-heeled black patent leather court shoes. She has a slightly nervous disposition and was always accompanied by her husband to her podiatry appointments. Her husband was always reported as being her 'rock' and undertook all the financial responsibilities of their married life.

Since Mrs Hilton's last appointment her husband suffered a short illness and died unexpectedly. As a result of this, her nervousness has been exacerbated and she is displaying signs of stress. Additionally, since Mrs Hilton's last appointment there has been a change in policy at the local Health Service Trust and she is no longer eligible for state-funded treatment. This situation has to be explained to her at her final appointment with the podiatrist.

PODIATRIC PRESENTATION

Mrs Hilton has cold, thin, bony feet, with bunions, lesser-toe deformity, corns and calluses. She has an uneventful medical history.

67

FACTORS INFLUENCING ENID'S BEHAVIOUR

Enid Hilton has just experienced the death of a loved one. Both the death and the events leading to it can have a range of physical and psychological effects and for some these can be devastating.

Mrs Hilton is in a state of confusion and feels extremely vulnerable at the loss of her long-time partner and friend. As a result of this she is demonstrating some of the signs of stress, reporting that she frequently cries and blames herself for her husband's death. She has feelings of being disempowered and out of control of her life.

Bereavement forces the bereaved person to accommodate significant changes, which can have a major impact on their social identity. In order for the podiatrist to help Mrs Hilton and to communicate with her effectively it is important to have an understanding of psychological impact of death and dying and also the stages associated with the bereavement process.

The processes of dying and death

Elderly people might be expected to be more accepting of death than younger people as they are more likely to have considered the possibility and even made preparations for the event. However, when death occurs unexpectedly, the impact may be more profound.

The anticipated loss of a partner can give rise to feelings of vulnerability that stem from fear and anger. Fear originates typically as a reaction to not being able to cope alone and the prospect of an unknown future. Anger can provide patients with a mechanism to cope with their grief but can also be destructive, especially when the aggression is directed towards members of the family and healthcare professionals. Anger is an understandable reaction and arises from feelings of intense personal frustration and the blocking of personal goals (Berkowitz 1993). However, Weiner (1986) points out that anger and aggression often stem from a sense of injustice and a belief that others are to blame. This is a common reaction and appears to reflect a fundamental human need to find an explanation for untoward events. Kubler-Ross (1969), in a

Table 8.1   Stages of dying (Kubler-Ross 1969)

Stage	Behavioural response
Denial	This is often the first reaction to being told the news that life is limited
Anger	The patient may try to blame others, including healthcare professionals
Bargaining	The patient may promise to change their behaviour, to be good or compliant or to give up bad habits in return for being able to live longer
Depression	If death is inevitable, the patient may become depressed and withdrawn and may refuse treatment. They may be anticipating their own death and mourning it
Acceptance	This is the final stage, where the patient is resigned and may wish to say farewell

seminal work based on studies of dying patients, challenged the taboo against discussing dying. This work helped to identify the needs of dying patients.

The process through which a bereaved person moves has been extensively described by Parkes (1986) as well as by Kubler-Ross (1969).

Kubler-Ross described five stages of dying (Table 8.1). These stages are not chronological and not all of the stages are experienced by all people.

Bereavement is the term describing the loss of a loved one; it is followed by a response that has been labelled the 'grief reaction'. Parkes (1972) studied widows in the first year of their bereavement and described the process as in Table 8.2. As with the process of dying, the stages are not fixed, but they are evident. Events and anniversaries are key times for the bereaved and may rekindle the grieving process.

The grief reaction includes emotions of fear, anger, guilt and sadness. Parkes (1972) argued that fear is caused by a sense of vulnerability and may result in the bereaved person avoiding the stressor that is causing the fear. Anger is caused by a sense of frustration and a belief that others are at fault, and may result in the bereaved person wanting to assign blame. Guilt is caused by a belief that the bereaved person has failed the person who has died. The bereaved person's reaction is to blame themselves.

Table 8.2 Stages of the grief reaction

Stage	Behavioural response
Denial	There may be feelings of numbness and a lack of reality. The bereaved person may cry a lot and feel that this is inappropriate behaviour. Mourning is a cultural expression of grief and will differ across different cultures
Yearning	The bereaved may want to hold on to personal items from the dead person such as clothing, letters or mementos
Despair	This may be intense and lead to depression. Widowed people may feel life is not worth living without their spouse
Recovery	This is gradual acceptance of the bereaved state, although some bereaved people report that 'you never get over it'

Intense sadness and feelings of emptiness are caused by the severance of attachment and the loss of an important part of self.

Although such models can oversimplify the process and experience of bereavement, they are useful to help understand the emotional stages that patients may experience.

Worden (1991) described the mechanisms of grief and the procedure for helping patients accomplish the 'tasks of mourning' to facilitate moving through the process. However, Ramsay & deGroot (1977) argued that the processes involved in coming to terms with loss might not be predictable in the staged way that theorists suggest. They proposed that there are nine components of grief, which may occur in different ways:

- Shock or numbness
- Disorganization or the lack of ability to plan
- Denial (expecting the spouse to return home)
- Depression
- Guilt at having neglected the spouse or treated him/her badly
- Anxiety about the future
- Aggression (towards doctors or family)
- Resolution or acceptance of the situation
- Re-integration into life.

Counsellors working with bereaved people also report that it is commonplace for the bereaved to see and or hear the person who has died, with remarkable realism.

The final stage of grief is recovery, although Stroebe et al (1993) suggest that complete recovery is often impossible. They propose that when 'there has been strong attachment to the lost one, involvement is likely to continue, even for a lifetime'.

Stroebe & Stroebe (1987) also suggest that the loss of a partner affects the survivor's social functioning in four main ways:

• Loss of social and emotional support
• Loss of social validation of personal judgements
• Loss of material and task supports – in most marriages there is role differentiation; after bereavement the survivor has to take on all roles
• Loss of social protection.

Difficulties in adjustment to being bereaved may also manifest in other ways. It is well established that a sharp increase in consultations with a general practitioner occurs following the death of a partner. There is also an increase in reported physical symptomatology among widowed people, accompanied by a 40% increase in mortality rate in the first 6 months following a spouse's death (Prigerson et al 1997).

Widowed people report behavioural problems with their children that Silverman & Worden (1993) ascribe to poor adjustment strategies by the surviving parent. Although there are several explanations for such findings, including reduction in immunocompetence, there are many who report that such symptoms and behaviours occur as a result of a 'broken heart'.

Challenge 1: Consider how you would inform Enid Hilton that she must be discharged

Mrs Hilton no longer qualifies for state-sector treatment. It is necessary for you to discharge her from your care. It is inevitable that the practitioner employed in the state sector will be subject to changes in funding arrangements as a result of political idiosyncrasies. These impact on the nature of the service that the podiatrist is able to provide, generally as reductions in the availability of care in real terms. The responsibility for implementing these policies and explaining the outcomes to patients falls to the practitioner.

1. Consider the impact of bereavement and the stages that individuals go through after a bereavement
2. Consider the boundaries between giving podiatric advice, general health advice and counselling
3. Consider how the involvement of others in the health, social work and voluntary sector teams may have a role in the care of bereaved people
4. Consider the needs of the podiatrist in this situation.

Challenge 2: What alternatives for support can be offered? What are the important psychological factors to be considered in Enid's case?

Enid has found her contact with the podiatrist to be very support-ive since her recent bereavement. Because of the new policy this contact will be terminated abruptly. What alternatives for support can be offered?

To be empowered is to have a good sense of identity and to feel that one has control over things that really matter. It also involves caring about others and feelings of belonging and of being accepted. Empowerment includes feeling being valued and being able to make a real contribution. Conversely, to feel disempowered is to feel insignificant, with a sense that life has little meaning, and to have little control over things that really matter. People with a low sense of empowerment may feel socially excluded and like an outsider in the society in which they live.

Stress can be said to be the result of a stressor, such as an adverse life event, which results in a response that has physical, emotional and behavioural components. Mrs Hilton is currently experiencing high levels of stress. This will make her more vul-nerable to the onset of illness. There is evidence that the immune system is compromised after prolonged periods of severe stress, and clearly Mrs Hilton is very vulnerable. Moreover, should she become ill, she will have greatly reduced resources to deal with her illness.

Early models of stress proposed by Seyle (1950) and Lazarus (1966) only considered physiological responses to stressors and did not examine the nature of stressors themselves. Cox (1978) later developed a transactional model of stress, in which he suggested that stress depends on the interaction between an individual and their environment. Cox proposed that the stress an individual experiences is the product of both the nature of the stressor and the individual's perception of their ability to cope with it. Perceived stress is therefore a highly subjective experience and different people will react differently to similar stressors.

This work has been echoed by Steptoe (1997), who proposed that: 'Stress responses are said to arise when demands exceed personal and social resources that the individual is able to mobilize'.

Coping resources and an individual's vulnerability (McEwan & Stellar 1993) are considered to be central to the relationship between stress and health. Predisposing biological and psychosocial factors and vulnerability play a dual role in the mechanism by which stress influences health. Physiological, behavioural and psychological processes may directly influence health in specific ways. For example, stress has measurable effects on the autonomic nervous system. Neuroendocrine mediators influence immune, gastrointestinal, neuromuscular and cardiovascular systems (McEwan 1998). Acute activation of these systems is known to precipitate short-term adaptive physiological changes as well as a whole range of somatic symptoms, which can manifest as increases in heart rate, perspiration and gastrointestinal motility. These symptoms may then be interpreted as indicative of illness.

Although physiological activation has short-term adaptive benefits, chronic activation of these systems is believed to enhance vulnerability to cardiovascular, metabolic, immune-related and other diseases (Chrousos & Gold 1992). In addition, such chronic activation results in changes in the central nervous system and brain (Sapolsky 1996). Behavioural responses such as changes in eating, sleeping and consumption of alcohol and other substances can increase the risk of illness and disease. Psychological symptoms also include altered self-perception and heightened awareness of body sensations. These sensations normally go unrecognized but may also be interpreted as indicators of illness (Pennebaker 1982).

The links between stress and ill-health have been questioned by some authors. In particular, it has been pointed out that many of the studies that demonstrate such a link have been retrospective in nature. This means that, while a clear association can be demonstrated to exist between stress and illness, data concerning stress and illness are gathered at the same time. Thus, while stress and illness co-occur, it is difficult to demonstrate that stress causes illness rather than the illness resulting in stress. In prospective studies, measures of stress are taken before illness occurs and are compared with illness at a later date. If a relationship is demonstrated in this way it would seem reasonable (although not certain) to conclude that stress is likely to cause illness rather than vice versa.

Such criticisms, however, may represent a simplistic approach in which stressful events are deemed to be the sole cause of disease rather than contributory factors that may alter *susceptibility* to disease (Dowrenwend et al 1982, Walker & Katon 1990).

ENID HILTON: SUMMARY OF IMPORTANT HEALTH PSYCHOLOGY

An understanding of the process of dying, death and bereavement are fundamental for the podiatrist to be able to respond to Mrs Hilton's needs. Reactions to actual or anticipated loss are complex and mediated by individual differences. Staged models are useful tools that help to explain the experiences of bereaved people. However, it is also important to recognize that not all such people will respond in the manner proposed by such models. Patients draw on their resources to cope with the trauma of bereavement. Such resources may include social support and the individual's characteristics, personality traits and habitual methods of dealing with stressful events.

The time taken for an individual to recover from bereavement varies widely and for most people the process is never truly complete. However, if acute grief persists longer than 18 months to

2 years it may be an indication that some form of help may be valuable. It is important for the podiatrist to recognize when such an intervention is necessary so that an appropriate referral can be made.

FURTHER READING

Cox T 1978 Stress. Macmillan, London
Kubler-Ross E 1993 On death and dying, 4th edn. Collier Books, New York
Parkes CM 1972 Bereavement: studies of grief in adult life. Penguin, Harmondsworth
Russell G 1999 Essential psychology for nurses and other health professionals. Routledge, London
Worden JW 1991 Grief counselling and grief therapy: handbook for the mental health practitioner, 2nd edn. Springer, New York

REFERENCES

Berkowitz A 1993 Aggression: its causes, consequences and control. McGraw-Hill, New York
Chrousos GP, Gold PW 1992 The concepts of stress and stress disorders. Overview of physical and behavioural homeostasis. Journal of the American Medical Association 267, 1244–1252
Cox T 1978 Stress. Macmillan, London
Dowrenwend B, Pearlin L, Clayton P et al 1982 Report on stress and life events. In: Elliott GR, Eisdorfer C (ed) Stress and human health: analysis and implications of research. Springer, New York, p. 55–80
Kubler-Ross E 1969 On death and dying. Tavistock, New York
Lazarus RS 1966 Psychological stress and coping process. McGraw-Hill, New York
McEwan BS 1998 Protective and damaging effects of stress mediators. New England Journal of Medicine 338, 171–179
McEwan BS, Stellar E 1993 Stress and the individual. Mechanisms leading to disease. Archives of Internal Medicine 153, 2093–2101
Parkes CM 1972 Bereavement: studies of grief in adult life. International University Press, New York
Parkes CM 1986 Bereavement: studies in grief in adult life, 3rd edn. Tavistock, London
Pennebaker J 1982 The psychology of physical symptoms. Springer, New York
Prigerson HG, Bierhals AJ, Kasel SV et al 1997 Traumatic grief as a risk factor for mental and physical morbidity. American Journal of Psychiatry 154, 616–623
Ramsay R, deGroot W 1977 A further look at bereavement. Paper presented at EATI conference Uppsala. Cited in Hodgkinson PE 1980 Treating abnormal grief in the bereaved. Nursing Times 76, 126–128
Sapolsky RM 1996 Why stress is bad for your brain. Science 273, 749–750
Seyle H 1950 Stress. Acta Medica, Montreal

Silverman PR, Worden JW 1993 Children's reactions to death of a parent. In Stroebe MS, Stroebe V Hansson RO (ed) Handbook of bereavement: theory, research and intervention. Cambridge University Press, Cambridge

Steptoe A 1997 Stress management. In Baum A, Newman S, Weinman J et al (ed) Cambridge handbook of psychology, health and medicine. Cambridge University Press, Cambridge

Stroebe W, Stroebe MS (1987) Bereavement and health: the psychological and physical consequences of partner loss. Cambridge University Press, New York

Stroebe MS, Stroebe W, Hansson RO 1993 Contemporary themes and controversies in bereavement research. In Stroebe MS, Stroebe V Hansson RO (ed) Handbook of bereavement: theory, research and intervention. Cambridge University Press, Cambridge

Walker EA, Katon WJ 1990 Psychological stress affecting physical conditions and responses to stress. In Stoudemire A (ed) Clinical psychiatry for medical students. JB Lippincott, Philadelphia, PA, p. 83–93

Weiner 1986 An attribution theory of motivation and emotion. Springer, New York

Worden JW 1991 Grief counselling and grief therapy: handbook for the mental health practitioner, 2nd edn. Springer, New York

9

Bill Canning – the relationship between socioeconomic status and health

Equality is the public recognition, effectively expressed in institutions and manners, of the principle that an equal degree of attention is due to the needs of all human beings.

Simone Weil

Bill is a 60-year-old school caretaker who is married and has four grown up children, all of whom have moved away from home. He lives in a two-bedroomed ex-council house which he has just finished buying. He works on a part-time basis at the local infant school where he has been employed for 10 years. The school has only a small number of children, is privately funded and is well maintained. Bill is shown little respect by the teaching staff and the headteacher is particularly patronizing towards him. However, the children love him and on the whole he enjoys his work.

Bill is an affable person and likes to socialize with his friends in the local pub. He is partial to 'a pint or two', especially on darts nights. Bill is a smoker who would not consider trying to give up because he believes that 'we all have to die from something'.

Bill is referred to the podiatrist with painful flat feet and bunions.

FACTORS THAT INFLUENCE BILL'S BEHAVIOUR

Bill's situation presents him with a dilemma. The lifestyle and behaviour that he adopts is different to that of the people who employ and work with him. There are times when he is made to feel uncomfortable as a result of this. There are thus three important issues to be considered in Bill's situation. First, the school is funded solely by fee-paying parents. As a result, paying for education and healthcare is viewed as a matter of individual choice, rather than state-funded education and healthcare being seen as a foundation of a just society. Moreover, there is strong support for the notion that paying for such services will result in them being 'better'.

Second, Bill is poorly paid in relation to the teaching staff and parents. He does not have the resources to exercise such 'choice'. Finally, Bill believes strongly that he has paid for his healthcare through taxation and that having to pay for such services is abdication of responsibility on the part of the state.

IMPORTANT PSYCHOLOGICAL THEORY

Socioeconomic status is a term used to describe a person's position in society, and is usually expressed in terms of income, education and occupation. It could also be represented by net worth, or by ownership of assets such as a home, car or other material possessions. By any such classification, Bill belongs to a lower socioeconomic group than his work colleagues and the children's parents.

The British population is generally more affluent than ever before. However, there is still little social mobility between the social classes. The most commonly used classification of socioeconomic status is that proposed by the Registrar General's classification of occupations. This framework classifies people according to their employment:

Class I – higher professional (e.g. medicine, law, architecture)
Class II – lower professional (e.g. nursing, podiatry, physiotherapy, management)
Class IIIn – skilled non-manual (e.g. secretarial workers, administrators)
Class IIIm – skilled manual (e.g. plumbers, electricians, mechanics)
Class IV – semiskilled workers (e.g. postmen, bus drivers, shop assistants)
Class V – unskilled labourers.

Minor modifications have been made to this scale from time to time, but it remains the method of classification used in the majority of British studies published in the past two decades.

It is important to note that this classification has a number of limitations. For example, in studies of families or couples the social class of the unit is generally defined by the occupation of the male partner. Secondly, some occupations in lower social groups are actually better paid than some found in higher groups.

There is much evidence that demonstrates that health status is unequal across different groups in British society (Townsend & Davidson 1982). Research suggests that health is related to geographical location, gender, age and socioeconomic status. For the last 30 years, it has been recognized that poorer people have poorer health than those who are better-off. Attention has been paid to this effect in the UK since the publication of the Black Report in 1980 (Townsend & Davidson 1982). Subsequent studies have demonstrated that this disparity in health status remains even when behavioural differences such as smoking, diet and physical activity are controlled. It is clear that there is a direct relationship between social deprivation and poorer health status (Beale 2001).

Other authors have examined the relationship between income and morbidity, both before and after controlling for other socioeconomic variables (Ecob & Davey Smith 1999). This study used data taken from the Health and Lifestyle National Survey of adults aged 18, which was conducted in 1984–5. It resulted in 9003 interviews being performed, which included questions concerning the material circumstances of the respondents. The results suggest that health is linearly related to income: *as income increases so health improves*. A further dimension to this is the size and quality of people's housing. Dunn & Hayes (2000) investigated two independent neighbourhoods in Vancouver. They found that both quality of housing and available living area per occupant were positively associated not only with socioeconomic status but also with health status. Dunn & Hayes (2000) also suggest that the circumstances of an individual's housing play an important role in determining their social status and social identity.

Other studies exist that demonstrate that a fear of illness and injury are much more common in patients from lower socio-economic classes (Noyes et al 2000). Moreover, there is evidence to suggest that people in such circumstances use healthcare services in a different way from those in higher socioeconomic groups. People of lower socioeconomic status receive less healthcare from the British National Health Service (NHS) than do those from higher socioeconomic classes (Le Grand 1980).

The NHS was originally set up to provide treatment free at the point of delivery irrespective of the patient's ability to pay. Although this ethic is still ostensibly maintained, there are occasions where either particular forms of healthcare fall outside the remit of the NHS or patients can expedite access to treatment by using the private sector. This has resulted in a situation that is quite different from the original concept of the NHS.

' The relationship between ability to pay for healthcare and the willingness to pay for it is complex and has been explored in only a few studies (Russell 1996, Donaldson 1999). However, this may become increasingly contentious as the nature of NHS provision changes in line with political thought.

The most common means of measuring inequalities in health status is known as the standardized mortality ratio (SMR). This is calculated as:

$$\frac{\text{The observed death rate in a given population} \times 100}{\text{The expected death rate in that population}}.$$

Thus a population that displays more deaths than would be expected has an SMR that is greater than 100 and a population that displays fewer deaths than would be expected has an SMR of less than 100. In all cases, the death rate may be controlled for the age distribution of the population. Over 20 years, the Black Report first demonstrated the SMR in the highest social class to be 77 for men and 82 for women, while the SMR in the poorest section of the population was 137 for men and 135 for women. It is known that this discrepancy has widened alarmingly since the publication of the Black Report.

Challenge 1: How can Bill best be treated, given that he has strongly held beliefs about private medicine?

You would like to refer Bill to a podiatric surgeon regarding surgical options for the treatment of his bunions, which are now extremely painful. This type of consultation is not available locally on the NHS. It would therefore be necessary for Bill to be seen in private practice. Bill is unable to afford the consultation fee or the costs of any subsequent surgery. He does not have any private medical insurance to cover these costs.

This scenario presents the podiatrist with a professional dilemma. It is a common reaction for professionals to be judgemental about how patients should prioritize their financial expenditure. It is clear that by curtailing his smoking and alcohol intake, Bill might be able to afford the necessary orthosis in a relatively short space of time. However, he is most reluctant to spend his money on private healthcare, believing that the NHS should provide him with any necessary treatment. In addition, he maintains that being a regular in his local pub represents 'his only pleasure'.

This problem reflects an important principle in understanding health-related behaviour. Risk to health is not always perceived as a deterrent to potentially damaging behaviours. It is very improbable that Bill is unaware of the risks that smoking and excessive drinking carry to his health. Many studies have demonstrated high levels of awareness of the risk of tobacco use among smokers (Vora et al 2000, Sasco & Kleihues 1999, Altman et al 1996). In fact, some research has shown that smokers may even overestimate the risks they run of developing certain diseases such as lung cancer (Sutton 1998).

However, Bill considers that these risks are worth taking because of the pleasure that he derives from his social life. Moreover, for many people immediate fulfilment is seen as preferable to benefits that are only accrued after a prolonged period of time.

The podiatrist has to make a decision as to whether to attempt to persuade Bill to change his behaviour in order to be able to afford surgery. Alternatively, it may be more appropriate simply to recognize Bill's needs while accepting that many patients may have values that are different to those of health professionals.

This is a matter for professional judgement and discretion, which can only be addressed adequately by understanding the patient as a whole and respecting and acknowledging their social identity, values and choices.

Challenge 2: How does the manner in which Bill is treated by his work colleagues influence his health and choices?

It is clearly established that inequalities in social status impact on physical health. However, it is equally important to appreciate that the British class system can be particularly destructive in terms of people's emotional health and sense of wellbeing.

People in lower socioeconomic groups are systematically made to feel disempowered and less valuable than those in higher socio-economic groups. Conversely, people in higher socioeconomic groups have their own sets of social constraints to which they are expected to conform. In Bill's case the offhand treatment he receives from his employers and the parents serves to foster his resentment against professionals in general. It is therefore possible that he may be less receptive to the podiatrist's well-meaning attempts to alter his smoking and drinking habits. In order to change Bill's behaviour, it is essential that he perceives any such change as being his choice rather than something that is imposed upon him. The podiatrist needs to understand this necessity and must develop a relationship of mutual trust and respect. The podiatrist's task is complete when s/he is assured that Bill is in receipt of all appropriate information in order to make an informed choice. However, Bill's choice may be at variance with that of the podiatrist and this must ultimately be accepted. Any attempt to change Bill's behaviour will rely heavily on the podiatrist possessing good communication skills, which underpin all podiatry practice.

BILL CANNING : SUMMARY OF IMPORTANT HEALTH PSYCHOLOGY

It is well established that substantial inequalities in health status are independently related to social status. People in lower socio-economic groups suffer from poorer health and have higher rates of mortality than people in higher socioeconomic groups. This effect is dependent upon *differences* in affluence rather than absolute measures of wealth. Western class systems equate social and financial position with intrinsic personal worth. Relative poverty thus results in the exclusion of less privileged people from complete participation in society.

FURTHER READING

Allot M, Robb M 1997 Health and social care. Sage, London
Beale N 2001 Unequal to the task: deprivation, health and UK general practice at the millennium. British Journal of General Practice 51, 584–585
Blaxter M 1990 Health and lifestyle. Routledge, London

REFERENCES

Altman DG, Levine DW, Coeytaux R et al 1996 Tobacco promotion and susceptibility to tobacco use among adolescents aged 12 through 17 years in a nationally representative sample. American Journal of Public Health 86, 1590–1593
Beale N 2001 Unequal to the task: deprivation, health and UK general practice at the millennium. British Journal of General Practice 51, 584–585
Donaldson C 1999 Valuing the benefits of publicly-provided health care: does 'ability to pay' preclude the use of willingness? Social Science and Medicine 49, 551–563
Dunn JR, Hayes MV 2000 Social inequality, population health and housing: a study of two Vancouver neighbourhoods. Social Science and Medicine 51, 563–587
Ecob R, Davey Smith G 1999 Income and health: what is the nature of the relationship? Social Science and Medicine 48, 693–705
Le Grand J 1980 The strategy of equality. Allen & Unwin, London
Noyes R Jr, Hartz AJ, Doebbeling CC et al 2000 Illness fears in the general population. Psychosomatic Medicine 62, 318–325
Russell S 1996 Ability to pay for health care: concepts and evidence. Health Policy and Planning 11, 219–237
Sasco AJ, Kleihues P 1999 Why can't we convince the young not to smoke? European Journal of Cancer 14, 1933–1940

Sutton S 1998 How ordinary people in Great Britain perceive the health risks of smoking. Journal of Epidemiology and Community Health 52, 338–339

Townsend P, Davidson N (ed) 1982 Inequalities in health. The Black report. Penguin Books, Harmondsworth

Vora AR, Yeoman CM, Hayter JP 2000 Alcohol, tobacco and paan use and understanding of oral cancer risk among Asian males in Leicester. British Dental Journal 188, 444–451

10

Olivia Saunders – working with children and their parents

How inimitably graceful children are in general before they learn to dance!

Samuel Taylor Coleridge

Olivia is an 8-year-old girl who has been having ballet lessons since she was 3 years of age. She has always loved dancing and already has aspirations to be a professional dancer. Her immediate ambition is to audition, as soon as possible, for a scholarship to the Royal Ballet School. She has worked hard at her ballet exams and has always passed with high marks and honours.

Olivia is a pretty young girl with a typical slim ballerina's physique. She is elegant and has poise with an air of determination and commitment when talking about her chosen career as a professional dancer. She is the only child of Mr and Mrs Saunders, who support their daughter and are very keen to help her to fulfil her ambition.

Olivia is pressurizing her parents to allow her to start to wear point shoes (ballet shoes with blocks in the toes) and to dance *en pointes*, even though she knows she is too young. She knows that she should really wait until she reaches menarche but feels that dancing *en pointes* will give her the edge over her peers. Olivia thinks that starting to wear point shoes will help her to achieve her goal of studying at the Royal Ballet School. Her ballet teacher, Miss Turner, would be very proud of Olivia if she were successful in achieving a scholarship and would see it as a direct reflection of her teaching ability. Miss Turner turned to teaching ballet after a disappointing career in the *corps de ballet* but always felt that her talents should have been recognized and that she was worthy of being a principal ballerina. She hopes to see Olivia have the acclaim that she never received. Mr and Mrs Saunders are influenced by the opinions of people they consider to be more expert than themselves. They have read that dancers should not be wearing point shoes as early as 8 years old, and need to be reassured that this is safe and appropriate before agreeing to Olivia's wishes. On the one hand they would like to accede to Olivia's demands but on the other hand they are concerned for her current and future health and welfare. Consequently, they have decided to seek impartial professional advice.

INFLUENTIAL FACTORS IN OLIVIA'S LIFE

Children do not think issues through in the same way as adults. Their thinking is simpler than that of adults and it is difficult for them to predict how an event or behaviour today might impact on tomorrow.

It is important to recognize that Olivia is very competitive and extremely motivated. Motivation is highly relevant to the achievement of the goals being pursued, to the intensity of the behaviour and to the persistence in the behaviour. Various early theories considered factors such as instinct, needs and drives but are now considered somewhat limited. For example, Maslow (1954, 1970) posited the existence of a 'hierarchy of needs' – shelter, food, etc. – that must be met for an individual to survive and to develop. These 'needs' provide motivational sources for behaviour. One aspect of motivation is the goal and the need of the individual to achieve that goal (Locke 1968). Locke suggested that there was a linear relationship between goal difficulty and level of performance. In Olivia's case, the goal is very difficult to achieve and will require high levels of performance, which may result in damage to her health.

Reinforcement is a technique that the podiatrist may employ with Olivia. Health professionals should provide positive reinforcement for behaviours that are most likely to help the patient achieve their goals. Patients seek both verbal and non-verbal positive feedback. Feedback expresses either approval of desired behaviour, or disapproval of maladaptive behaviour.

Another approach to consider is the use of positive role models. Identification with a positive role model can demonstrate positive health values and outcomes.

Children who have positive role models around them, or who identify with positive role models, are more likely to chose the same healthy behaviours. This may in turn provide a positive self-image that remains with the child throughout life (Ikeda & Naworski 1992).

Olivia needs to be aware that she may become subject to ankle and foot injury as a result of excessive training. Acute traumatic injuries are common in ballet dancers (MacIntyre & Joy 2000). Where there is incomplete rehabilitation, they often develop into repeated injuries.

Cuboid subluxations in females differ from those occurring in males (Marshall & Hamilton 1992, MacIntyre & Joy 2000). In men, cuboid dislocations are usually acute and occur as a result of a series of jumps (in ballet terms – a 'bravura' variation) when the foot is repeatedly pronated under force. A sequence of movements such as *relevés* (a repetitive movement from foot flat to balancing on the tips of the toes, and back again) can result in overuse syndrome. Dancers moving from foot flat to 'full point' (on the tips of their toes) may find remaining in the full point position difficult and consequently balance on the dorsal surface of the metatarsal heads. In addition, the resultant alterations of direction and force applied to the foot during repetitive movements such as *relevés* will contribute to reduced joint stability. The repetitive nature of ballet movements can result in hypermobility, which in turn predisposes dancers to cuboid dislocations (Marshall & Hamilton 1992, MacIntyre & Joy 2000). While it is possible for females to dislocate the cuboid, subluxation of the cuboid is more common and a result of overuse; it may become part of an 'overuse syndrome'.

Ligamentous laxity is considered as a further factor in the cause of dance injury (Newell & Woodie 1981, Blakeslee & Morris 1987, Marshall & Hamilton 1992, MacIntyre & Joy 2000). Most ballet dancers subject their joints to extreme ranges of movement in order to perform certain sequences, thereby increasing the likelihood of injury (Newell & Woodie 1981, Blakeslee & Morris 1987, Marshall & Hamilton 1992, MacIntyre & Joy 2000).

Comprehensive assessment, diagnosis and management of acute injury is required to prevent injuries such as ligament tears and tendon pathologies from becoming chronic. As part of management, attention should be paid to nutrition in order both to facilitate healing of existing injuries and to prevent the possible development of conditions such as osteoporosis. Osteoporosis is considered in more detail in the case of *Suzi Dalton* (Chapter 4). Without consideration of the psychological factors associated with injury, pain perception and concordance with treatment, successful rehabilitation may be limited.

Great care should be exercised when designing a training regime for prepubescent children. Growth periods are difficult to identify and are of uncertain duration. Therefore no undue pressure should be placed on the long bones when epiphyseal closure may not have taken place. Moreover, submaximal muscle strength training is more appropriate to the growing child. This involves the use of training that focuses on the trunk and is considered to provide flexibility, balance and coordination, which are fundamental to remaining injury-free (Phillips 1999). Such a training regime is preferable to the early use of point shoes and the podiatrist should suggest this approach to Olivia and her parents.

The presence of painful skin lesions (e.g. corns) and in particular interdigital lesions, often results in dancers suspending their training regime. Golomer & Chatellier (1990) found that the number of skin lesions is correlated to the degree of tightness of the point shoe – the tighter the shoe, the more skin lesions. Palliative podiatric treatment, in other words the reduction of the painful corns, will allow dancers to return to their training schedule; however, it is almost inevitable that the lesions will recur and disrupt training once again.

In addition to skin, other soft tissue structures such as tendons, bursae and fascia may be injured as a consequence of excessive and repeated stress. Finally, joint injury may result in longer periods of rehabilitation, with recurring episodes of injury responsible for chronic joint disease leading, in the long term, to arthritis.

It is a truism, but important, to consider that the tips of the toes were never intended to support the entire body weight and that such an abnormal posture will inevitably result in pain and injury.

Challenge 1: What are the possible motivations for Olivia's wish to wear point shoes?

Such factors might include:

- Competitiveness
- A desire to be 'grown-up'
- A desire and/or need to be the first in her group to achieve desired goals
- The normal inability of children to assess the long-term effects of present behaviour
- A desire to please her dance teacher.

You should consider this challenge and reflect on how you would feel if asked to offer an opinion regarding the wisdom of Mr and Mrs Saunders allowing Olivia to dance *en pointes*. It is likely that what you have to say will not be what Olivia wishes to hear, and she may resent your involvement. You will have to consider how you can deliver this information in a way that will be acceptable to Olivia.

Challenge 2: How can you enable both Olivia and Mr and Mrs Saunders to acknowledge the benefits of not progressing yet to point shoes?

The information that Olivia requires includes the importance, from both a developmental and a foot health perspective, of her not wearing point ballet shoes until at least her menarche. Structurally her feet are not yet strong enough to be able to deal with stresses of dancing *en pointes* and she has a greater chance of developing toe deformities.

A useful approach to health promotion might involve:

- Exploring Olivia's beliefs about early point work
- Reinforcing any positive attitudes she may have
- Discussing myths and attitudes towards dance
- Exploring with Olivia and her parents the perceived costs and benefits of dancing *en pointes*
- Providing reliable information to assist the family to make informed choices
- Devising a negotiated plan of action
- Monitoring Olivia's progress.

The health education and promotion approach could include the use of strengthening exercises, which would prepare Olivia for the time when she reaches a suitable age to wear point shoes. If possible, alternatives to wearing point shoes should also be suggested. This approach may provide different positive reinforcement for Olivia. It will also provide Mr and Mrs Saunders with an explanation of the short- and long-term costs and benefits if Olivia chooses to dance *en pointes* early.

OLIVIA SAUNDERS: SUMMARY OF IMPORTANT HEALTH PSYCHOLOGY

It is important that the podiatrist understands the complex interactions that can occur between a professional, a child and the child's parent/s. Well-developed interpersonal and communication skills are essential to assure a successful outcome in a situation such as this. An understanding of effective health promotion is important in order to design strategies that will enable Olivia to prevent the development of injuries.

FURTHER READING

Hagins M (ed) 2002 Dance medicine resource guide, 2nd edn. J Michael Ryan, Andover, NJ
Brinson P 1996 Fit to dance? The report of the national inquiry into dancers' health. Calouste Gulbenkian Foundation, London

REFERENCES

Blakeslee TJ, Morris JL 1987 Cuboid syndrome and the significance of midtarsal joint stability. Journal of the American Podiatric Medical Association 77, 12

Golomer E, Chatellier K 1990 Anthropometrie du pied du chausson de pointe et pathologie cutanée. Cinesiologie 29, 277–282

Ikeda J, Naworski P 1992 Am I fat? Helping young children accept differences in body size. ETR Associates, Santa Cruz, CA

Locke EA 1968 Toward a theory of task motivation and incentives. Organisational Behaviour and Human Performance 3, 157–189

MacIntyre J, Joy E 2000 The athletic woman – foot and ankle injuries in dance. Clinics in Sports Medicine 19, 351–368

Marshall MA, Hamilton WG 1992 Cuboid subluxations in ballet dancers. American Journal of Sports Medicine 20, 2

Maslow AH 1954 Motivation and personality. Harper, New York

Maslow AH 1970 Towards a psychology of being. Van Nostrand, New York

Newell SG, Woodie A 1981 Cuboid syndrome. Physician and Sports Medicine 9, 71–76

Phillips C 1999 Strength training of dancers during the adolescent growth spurt. Journal of Dance Medicine and Science 3, 66–72

11

Peter Brennan – dealing with sensitive and confidential material

It is tact that is golden, not silence.

Samuel Butler

Peter Brennan is 35 years old. He is a small man approximately 1.7 m tall and weighs about 60 kg. Peter has a serious face, dark eyes and dark brown hair and looks slightly older than his actual age. He is employed as a social worker by the local authority, in a senior position. Apart from his podiatric condition, he seems fit and well, with a cheerful, open manner. As part of taking his history, the podiatrist asks him whether he is taking any form of medication. Peter replies that he has been on continuous combined therapy since being diagnosed as positive for human immunodeficiency virus (HIV) 3 years ago. He has remained well throughout this period and is in regular contact with local HIV services. While he is direct about his condition in the context of his treatment, Peter does not make his HIV status known generally. Peter is single and lives alone in a flat in a pleasant part of the town. He has a sister who lives at the other end of the country. Peter's parents, although elderly, are both alive and well; his relationship with them is good.

PODIATRIC PRESENTATION

Peter presents with multiple warts on the plantar surface of his feet. The podiatrist wants to use an antiviral, which is a prescription-only medicine, and it will therefore be necessary for the podiatrist to contact Peter's GP. It is extremely important that Peter's lesions are kept free from possible infection following treatment.

Patients who are immunosuppressed are more susceptible to secondary infections, which they are less able to overcome.

Clearly Peter's HIV status presents a number of problems in relation to infection control. These may be usefully considered first in relation to himself and second in relation to those professionals providing his treatment. Patients whose immune systems are compromised for any reason, including HIV infection, are much more susceptible to secondary infection and this must be taken into consideration when considering Peter's treatment regime.

HUMAN IMMUNE DEFICIENCY VIRUS INFECTION

Causes and risks of human immune deficiency virus infection

Viral infection with HIV gradually destroys the immune system. Acute HIV infection may be associated with symptoms resembling mononucleosis (glandular fever) or flu within 2–4 weeks of exposure. HIV seroconversion (changing from being HIV-negative to HIV-positive) occurs within 3 months of exposure.

People who become infected with HIV may have no symptoms for up to 10 years, but they can still transmit the infection to others. Meanwhile, their immune system gradually weakens until they are diagnosed with acquired immune deficiency syndrome (AIDS). Acute HIV infection progresses over time to asymptomatic HIV infection and then to early symptomatic HIV infection and later, to AIDS.

HIV infection may be passed through the maternal blood-stream to the fetus, resulting in the baby being HIV-positive when born. HIV may also be transmitted by contact with infected blood, and frequently occurs when intravenous drug users share injecting equipment. More commonly, HIV is transmitted sexually. Although the infection was first noticed in the 1980s among gay men, heterosexually transmitted HIV infection is now much more common and is increasing rapidly.

Most individuals infected with HIV progress to AIDS if not treated. However, there is a very small subset of patients who develop AIDS very slowly or never at all. These patients are called non-progressors.

Acquired immune deficiency syndrome

AIDS is caused by HIV. It is characterized by the progressively immunocompromised state of the infected individual (Soltani et al 1996). Disease progression is monitored by a continuous decrease in peripheral blood CD4+ T lymphocytes, which are targeted by HIV infection. These cells play an important role in the immune system, hence the gradual loss of the patient's immune defences. AIDS is the final and most serious stage of HIV disease, in which the signs and symptoms of severe immune deficiency have developed.

Cutaneous podiatric implications

The course of HIV can have a devastating effect on lower limb mobility and function and the role of the podiatrist may be fundamental to the care team (McReynolds 1995). Podiatrists will be particularly aware of the opportunistic infections occurring as a result of cell-mediated and humoral immunodeficiency. The most common infections are caused by *Staphylococcus aureus*, beta-haemolytic streptococci from groups A, C and G and *Pseudomonas aeruginosa* (Memar et al 1995). Furthermore, in the early stages of the disease tinea pedis (fungal infections) and verrucas are more common. Smith et al (1994) report that verrucas appeared to become more diffuse and resilient to treatment as the disease progressed. Other complications include increased risk of cutaneous epidermal and melanotic malignancies, including Kaposi's sarcoma. Non-infectious disorders include inflammatory disorders, pruritus, hypersensitivities, dryness and dermatoses.

Challenge 1: What are the important issues concerning Peter's psychological care?

It is very important to appreciate that adequate protection against accidental infection with HIV is afforded by routine procedures, often described as 'universal precautions'. Such procedures are those that should be taken with all patients, not just Peter, and the podiatrist does not need to take any other specific precautions when treating a patient who is known to be HIV-positive. In Peter's case any of the available treatments may involve the use of debridement, which could result in loss of some blood or serous fluid. However, such clinical waste should always be treated with appropriate care because many patients may be carrying blood-borne diseases of which they are unaware, some of which (e.g. viral hepatitis) are far more contagious than HIV. Much unnecessary fear and misunderstanding continues to exist with regard to HIV transmission, even among health professionals. Such misunderstanding may easily manifest in levels of caution that are inappropriate and can serve to distance still further patients who already experience prejudice and alienation as a result of the public reaction to their condition.

Nevertheless, there are important issues for the podiatrist concerning Peter's treatment. It must be recognized that consideration of the route by which Peter acquired the virus is outside the professional boundaries of podiatric practice and is irrelevant to his podiatric treatment. All podiatrists, like other health professionals, have a *duty of care*, which requires them to provide treatment to the best of their ability. In order to achieve this with all patients, it is insufficient for podiatrists to assume that their duty of care negates any discriminatory feelings they may hold. There will be times when patients present information that is contrary to the podiatrist's beliefs or culture. It is necessary for the podiatrist to recognize not only that such differences will occur but also that all people are free to behave and express themselves in a manner that is appropriate for them. It is also very important for practitioners to recognize their own professional boundaries and not to attempt to address issues that are outside their scope of practice and competence. All health professionals must therefore examine their attitudes toward complex issues such as drug use and sexuality in relation to their own professional practice.

The need for confidentiality is particularly important in Peter's treatment. While confidentiality is an essential characteristic of all patient–therapist interactions, the emotive response sometimes generated by HIV-related issues has specific implications for his welfare. Peter works in the public sector in a sensitive position that is often the subject of criticism and stereotyping (Pietroni 1991). Confidentiality is a fundamental right of all patients and in Peter's case unauthorized disclosure of his status could be extremely damaging.

However, the podiatrist will need to contact Peter's GP for prescription of the antiviral medication and possible onward referral to dermatology. This may raise issues of confidentiality because the GP may not necessarily be aware of Peter's HIV status. It will be necessary to negotiate permission for this dialogue.

Challenge 2: What are the particular needs of Peter in relation to his podiatric condition?

Recent research (James et al 2001) has shown that patients taking combination therapy are more prone to onychocryptosis or ingrowing toe nails. James and colleagues found that, out of a group of 74 patients taking indinavir and ritonavir, five patients (6.8%) were suffering from onychocryptosis involving the big toe. Onychocryptosis is often associated with paronychia (inflammation of the skin surrounding the nails), which may lead to infection. While such infections are easily treated in most patients, people with HIV have suppressed immune systems and minor infections can become much more serious in a short space of time. It is therefore very important that any signs of infection are dealt with without delay.

James et al (2001) stress that, as combination therapy becomes more widely used, complications such as ingrowing toe nails are more likely to become more common. The authors further recommend that all patients taking combination therapy should have their hands and feet examined regularly.

PETER BRENNAN: SUMMARY OF IMPORTANT ISSUES

There are four key issues in relation to Peter's podiatric treatment and management.

• The spread of HIV infection is adequately controlled by the use of universal precautions and no special procedures are required over and above those of normal hygiene and cross-infection control protocols

• It is important for the podiatrist to recognize his/her professional competence in relation to Peter's infection

• Confidentiality is an essential part of the care of any patient but the nature of Peter's condition brings the need for confidentiality into sharper focus

• It is very important, when treating patients who are immunosuppressed in any way, to conduct a thorough examination for signs of infection so that treatment can be instigated at the earliest opportunity.

REFERENCES

James CW, McNeils KC, Cohen DM et al 2001 Recurrent ingrown toenails secondary to indinavir/ritonavir combination therapy. Annals of Pharmacotherapy 35, 881–884

McReynolds M 1995 Rehabilitation management of the lower extremity in HIV disease. Journal of the American Podiatric Medical Association 85, 394–401

Memar O, Cirelli R, Lee P, Tyring S 1995 Cutaneous manifestations of HIV-1 infection. Journal of the American Podiatric Medical Association 85, 362–373

Pietroni PC 1991 Stereotypes or archetypes? A study of perceptions amongst health-care students. Journal of Social Work Practice 5, 61–69

Smith K, Skelton H, Yeager J, et al and the Military Medical Consortium for the Advancement of Retroviral Research (MMCARR) 1994 Cutaneous findings in HIV-1 positive patients: a 42-month prospective study. Journal of the American Academy of Dermatology 31, 746–753

Soltani S, Kenyon E, Barbosa P 1996 Chronic and aggressive plantar verrucae in a patient with HIV. Journal of the American Podiatric Medical Association 86, 555–558

12

Harriet Edmondson – an adolescent with a suspected eating disorder

If I talk, everyone thinks I'm showing off; when I'm silent they think I'm ridiculous; rude if I answer, sly if I get a good idea, lazy if I'm tired, selfish if I eat a mouthful more than I should, stupid, cowardly, crafty, etc. etc.

Anne Frank

Harriet is a 15-year-old who is referred to your practice with an ingrowing toe nail. She is tall and slim and is wearing loose sports-wear consisting of track-suit bottoms and an over-large sweat shirt. Harriet has a thin face with high cheek bones. These are accentuated by the fact that Harriet has her long hair swept back tightly into a pony tail, which makes her look rather severe. The podiatrist has just completed an evening class in personal coun-selling and as a result has become quite observant of the patients' non-verbal behaviour. The podiatrist notices that Harriet is a reserved girl with a sullen facial expression, which does not change when she engages in conversation. She avoids making eye contact with anyone and appears to be reticent, withdrawn and rather intense. Harriet reports that her ingrowing toe nail occurred as a result of a netball accident in which her opponent accidentally jumped and landed on her toe. Initially the toe was inflamed and the nail was torn and ragged. Harriet reports that 'it felt like it had something sticking in it' and so she tried to 'tidy up' the nail with her nail scissors. Harriet reports that she plays netball twice a week at school and is also a member of a local team. When she is not playing netball she also likes to keep fit by using the gym at her mother's sports club.

Harriet is accompanied by her mother, who is extremely smart and is wearing a well-cut business suit with expensive jewellery. She has an air of efficiency but a rather patronizing conversation style. She is clearly irritated by her daughter's action to self-treat, which has resulted in this injury. She has been forced to take time off work to bring her daughter to the clinic for professional help. Conversation between Harriet and her mother is limited.

PODIATRIC PRESENTATION

Harriet is reluctant to let the podiatrist inspect her toe and is adamant that no-one may touch it. Having been coaxed into removing her trainer and sock, she presents a first toe nail that is extremely red, swollen and oozing thick, yellow pus. The sides of the toe are bulging and have exuded over the nail plate leaving only a small amount of nail plate exposed. While she is indicating the point where the nail seems to be digging in, the podiatrist notices that she has very bitten finger nails and that the skin around the nails has been picked, leaving the tissue raw and inflamed.

FACTORS THAT INFLUENCE HARRIET'S BEHAVIOUR

Harriet likes competition and competing: she says it makes her feel good and gives her a 'buzz'. She is a serious athlete and maintenance of fitness and her figure are extremely important to her. For a girl of 15 her face and overall physique appear to be extremely thin. However, it is difficult to assess this fully because the type of clothing she has chosen to wear covers her arms and legs completely. She seems nervous and picks at her fingers when not engaged in conversation.

Adolescence is the stage that represents the transition between childhood and adulthood and an understanding of adolescent behaviour is important. Adolescence is a phase marked by significant physical changes including altered body shape. In addition, body image becomes more important, cognitive development accelerates and relations with adults, parents and authority may become difficult. It is also a time of uncertainty, when decisions are made in relation to future careers and developments.

Marcia (1966) proposes the notion of an adolescent identity crisis, or a time when adolescents have no sense of a personal identity and which is characterized by strong feelings of uncertainty. Marcia also suggests that adolescents tend to move from low identity status to high identity status as a result of growing external and internal pressures on them to enter the adult world. Erikson (1968) identifies stages in adolescent development and suggests that adolescence is a time when individuals strive to avoid role confusion. Adolescents use peer groups to develop a sense of social identity. Waterman (1982) notes that adolescents who had affectionate parents who gave them sufficient freedom to become individuals in their own right tended to have explored and considered different alternatives for themselves. By contrast, adolescents whose parents were domineering were less likely to have considered their own identity, while adolescents whose parents were aloof and uninvolved tended neither to have considered their identity nor to have any commitment to the future (Waterman 1982).

While Harriet exhibits many typical features of adolescence, she also shows signs that would lead the podiatrist to suspect that all was not well.

Peer pressure is acknowledged to be highly influential during the adolescent period. At adolescence, peer relations expand to occupy a particularly central role in young people's lives. New types (e.g. opposite-sex, romantic ties) and levels (e.g. 'crowds') of peer relationships emerge. Peers typically replace the family as the centre of a young person's socializing and leisure activities. Teenagers have multiple peer relationships, and they confront multiple 'peer' cultures that have remarkably different norms and value systems.

Peers can have extremely powerful influence in the teenage years. Estimates suggest that around one in six adolescents are bullied. Teenagers may be bullied by their peers for a number of reasons, including:

- Appearance, such as being overweight
- Resisting the pressure to conform

* Background, including race and socioeconomic factors
* Academic achievement.

It is therefore important that vulnerable adolescents are provided with appropriate support in order to cope with such difficulties. Research suggests that friendships are very important to young people's overall growth, stability and personal development. Friends provide social and cognitive skills for each other that would otherwise be lacking. Having friends has been proved to show positive outcomes in both boys and girls, and across different cultural groups and different intelligence levels (Bukowski et al 1996).

Behavioural characteristics, attitudes and the qualitative features of these relationships are all important factors in predicting the developmental outcomes of the friendships (Bukowski et al 1996). While peer influence is neither good nor bad as a whole, it can go either way very easily, depending on the adolescents and the group, as well as the dynamics that take place within it.

Pre-adolescent children spend far less time with their friends and more time being monitored by adults, often their parents. Less time with other children, and more parental direction, makes for less peer influence. By contrast, adolescents seek less time with adults and more with peers. In the process of forming an independent identity, adolescents are relatively easily influenced as they seek their independence.

In general, most adolescents tend to follow similar paths to their independence. However, the presence of a few poorly adjusted individuals may have a profound influence on group behaviour. Pearson & Michell (2000) describe a process of 'deviancy training' within some adolescent friendships that results in increases in delinquency, substance use, violence and adult maladjustment.

The adolescent period is also a time when anorexia nervosa can develop. Anorexia nervosa is an eating disorder that is thought to develop as a coping mechanism to both external and internal influences and conflicts. People with anorexia usually have a perception of being overweight and a heightened sensitivity to and fear of becoming fat. Anorexia nervosa is often associated with low self-esteem and the need for acceptance. It occurs primarily in adolescent females (12–25 years), and more commonly in families from higher socioeconomic groups. Anorexia nervosa is 20 times more prevalent among females than males. Among ballet dancers the prevalence may be as high as 3.5–7.6% (Nelson 1996).

The most common features of anorexia nervosa are loss of weight, coupled with changes in behaviour. The weight loss is slowly progressive and often follows on from a weight-reducing diet. It is only after several months that it becomes clear that the dieting is pathological and the weight loss extreme. Initially, weight loss may be positively reinforced by favourable comments by friends and family about the individual's new, slimmer appearance. However, as the weight loss continues, attempts to challenge the sufferer's further dieting are usually met with anger, deceit or a combination of both. Often, families are ill-equipped to deal with this situation and may resort to confrontation, bullying or bribery, all of which usually fail.

Increasing introversion manifests in the sufferer becoming less outgoing, less sociable and less fun. Contact with friends may be lost and a lack of interest in everything apart from the avoidance of food and increased commitment to academic work often becomes apparent. The person with anorexia may also display obsessional behaviour, especially in relation to food and to exercise. This may be observed in the fastidious weighing of food, drinking abnormally large volumes of water, and a marked increase in the intensity and duration of exercise. Excessive exercise is frequently observed in people with anorexia nervosa and has been considered to be both an addiction and an obsessive compulsive disorder under these circumstances (Davis et al 1999). Loss of confidence and assertiveness are often seen in people suffering from anorexia, who may also become less argumentative and more dependent on others. At the same time their anorexic behaviour will increasingly control the lives of those close to them.

The causes of anorexia nervosa appear to be multifactorial. Factors may include personality, aspects of family members and relationships within the family. External stresses and problems and problems with friendships at school are often factors in the aetiology. The increased incidence of anorexia nervosa in families where there are other anorexics may indicate a genetic predisposition.

People predisposed to anorexia tend to be conformist, compliant and hard-working. They are often popular with teachers and may appear to given little cause for worry over the years. As their contemporaries go through the difficulties of adolescence they seem models of sensible behaviour by comparison. These traits may be quite marked before the onset of anorexia but they are usually accentuated by the disorder.

Osteoporosis and amenorrhoea are symptoms of a hormonal imbalance brought about by anorexia nervosa (Nishizawa et al 2001). This is because the disorder not only interrupts the normal rapid bone accretion characteristics of adolescents but also accelerates bone loss. Low body mass and low calcium intake contribute further to the risk of osteoporosis.

Harriet may see the podiatrist as an establishment figure, which could create difficulties in establishing a relationship. Paton & Brown (1991) suggest that health professionals communicating with adolescents require a sensitive approach in order that they are not perceived as a 'parent'. Often, discussions of a personal nature are particularly embarrassing for adolescents and they may be reluctant to reveal their anxieties for fear of being considered 'silly'. All adolescents feel particularly self-conscious about their bodies, and podiatrists need to ensure that adolescent patients feel confident that their privacy and confidentiality are guaranteed.

Challenge 1: What should the podriatist do about Harriet's suspected anorexia nervosa?

You suspect that Harriet may be suffering from anorexia nervosa. You have also attended a part-time counselling course in which eating disorders were discussed. Is Harriet's suspected condition an issue that you should address?

Anorexia nervosa is a condition whose aetiology is complex and not always well understood. Its treatment is difficult and not always successful. It is very unlikely that the podiatrist will have the experience, skills or time necessary to intervene in Harriet's case and it is important that s/he is cognizant of the limits of her/his professional competence. However, it may be very difficult for podiatrists to ignore the natural desire to help. If this is the case, then any approach should be made confidentially through Harriet's mother as Harriet is likely to be defensive about her eating behaviour. This is complicated in Harriet's case, as her relationship with her mother appears to be strained. It should also be noted that Harriet is below the age of consent for medical treatment should any referral be considered.

The presentation of the toe nail indicates that Harriet may need a minor surgical procedure. As the nail is so painful this will require the careful administration of an injection of local anaesthetic to block pain sensation.

Consider how you would deliver this information to Harriet.

Challenge 2: What psychological issues should the podiatrist consider prior to performing any surgical procedure?

Kitshore (1999) reported on preoperative anxiety and patient's information needs, and the findings are consistent with the much larger nursing literature in which the physical and psychological needs of patients undergoing elective day surgery (Mitchell 1997, Calvin & Lane 1999), and in particular the needs of children experiencing day surgery (Murphy Taylor 1999), are considered.

Miller (1980) suggests that patients awaiting surgery may act in one of two ways with regard to their desire for information. Those she calls 'monitors' seek out as much information as possible concerning their condition and its treatment in order reduce their anxiety. By contrast, those Miller describes as 'blunters' prefer not to know what is to happen to them and avoid such information as much as possible. Patients who are 'monitors' are thus likely to find the delivery of preoperative information beneficial in reducing anxiety. However, patients who are 'blunters' may find that such information raises their anxiety.

It may be helpful for some patients undergoing minor surgery under local anaesthetic to be given some control over the procedure in order to reduce their anxiety. Taylor (1986) suggests that there are four kinds of control involved:

- **Behavioural control** involves the patient being able to control the progress of a procedure in some way and this reduces anxiety, for example an agreement is made such as that the procedure will stop on a predetermined signal from the patient such as raising a hand
- **Cognitive control** involves the use of distraction techniques to concentrate the patient's thoughts on things other than the procedure, for example the use of relaxing music
- **Decision control** involves the patient having some influence over when they are ready and wish to have the procedure performed
- The effectiveness of **information control** is illustrated in the case of Miller's (1980) 'monitors', who find the provision of information reassuring.

Harriet's general health is a cause for concern. She is currently debilitated through malnutrition and her healing ability is likely to be compromised. Your management of this should thus include arranging the provision of antibiotic therapy from her GP. It will be necessary for the podiatrist to obtain Harriet's and her mother's consent to approach Harriet's doctor to ensure that there are no contraindications to the surgery.

The provision of information for post-operative care is important for patients undergoing nail surgery. For Harriet, this advice will involve her stopping her exercise routine temporarily. This is likely to be difficult for her and will require skill and tact on the part of the podiatrist.

HARRIET EDMONDSON: SUMMARY OF IMPORTANT PSYCHOLOGICAL FACTORS

Adolescence is always a period characterized by emotional instability. Adolescents may be volatile in their relationships with adults in general, and their parents in particular. Anorexia is an uncommon but potentially extremely serious condition, which requires specialist intervention. It is essential for health professionals to be aware of and work within the limitations of their own competence and scope of practice. It is also important for practitioners to restrict their practice to that of the context in which they are working.

FURTHER READING

Heaven P 2001 The social psychology of adolescence. Macmillan, Basingstoke
Orford J 2001 Excessive appetites: a psychological view of addiction. Jossey-Bass, San Francisco, CA

REFERENCES

Bukowski WM, Newcomb AF, Hartup WW 1996 The company they keep: friendship in childhood and adolescence. Cambridge University Press, New York
Calvin RL, Lane PL 1999 Perioperative uncertainty and state anxiety of orthopaedic surgical patients. Orthopaedic Nursing 18, 61–66
Davis C, Katzman DK, Kirsh C 1999 Compulsive physical activity in adolescents with anorexia nervosa: a psychobehavioural spiral of pathology. Journal of Nervous and Mental Diseases 187, 336–342
Erikson EH 1968 Identity, youth and crisis. Norton, New York
Kitshore A 1999 Information needs and anxiety in patients anticipating toe nail surgery. British Journal of Podiatry 2, 108–118
Marcia J 1966 Development and validation of ego-identity status. Journal of Personality and Social Psychology 3, 551–558
Miller SM 1980 When is a little information a dangerous thing? Coping with stressful events by monitoring and blunting. In Levine S, Ursin H (ed) Coping and health. Plenum Press, New York
Mitchell M 1997 Patients' perceptions of pre-operative preparation for day surgery. Journal of Advanced Nursing 26, 356–363
Murphy Taylor C 1999 Children's nursing. The benefits of preparing children and parents for day surgery. British Journal of Nursing 8, 801–804
Nelson DP 1996 Validity concerns in previous studies examining the frequency of anorexia nervosa in ballet dancers. Microform Publications, International Institute for Sport and Human Performance, University of Oregon, Eugene, OR
Nishizawa K, Iijima M, Tokita A, Yamashiro Y 2001 Bone mineral density of eating disorder. Nippon Rinsho/Japanese Journal of Clinical Medicine 59, 554–560
Paton D, Brown R 1991 Lifespan health psychology: nursing problems and interventions. Harper Collins, London

Pearson M, Michell L 2000 Smoke rings: social network analysis of friendship groups, smoking and drug-taking. Drugs Education Prevention and Policy 7, 21–37

Taylor SE 1986 Health psychology. Random House, New York

Waterman AS 1982 Identity development from adolescent to adulthood. An extension of theory and review research. Developmental Psychology 18, 341–348

13

Margaret Knowles – the conflict between medical and social needs

> *The Family is the Country of the heart. There is an angel in the Family who, by the mysterious influence of grace, of sweetness, and of love, renders the fulfilment of duties less wearisome, sorrows less bitter.*
>
> Giuseppe Mazzini

Margaret is a 60-year-old woman who lives in a one-bedroom flat on the 16th floor of a tower block. The block of flats was built in the 1960s and has a dreary appearance, being constructed from concrete. The area demonstrates little architectural attractiveness. The ground floor is defaced by graffiti and the lift is regularly out of order. The few shops nearby that are still trading have metal shuttering erected at night to prevent vandalism. The local community has few facilities and has neither a health centre nor a community centre. Unemployment rates are above average and the older local residents are fearful about being out in the streets after dark.

Mrs Knowles lives alone, having been widowed 15 years ago. She has a daughter, a lone parent, who lives in a nearby block of flats with her two children. Mrs Knowles helps to look after her grandchildren, enabling her daughter to work part-time and also to have an occasional break from child care. Mrs Knowles works as a shelf stacker in the local convenience store. She likes the flexibility of the work, which enables her to pick up her grandchildren after school every day. Every fourth week she takes the opportunity of visiting the podiatrist, whose surgery is in the centre of town and close to her grandchildren's school. The children attend the Roman Catholic primary school, which is located approximately

10 minutes walk from the podiatrist's surgery. Mrs Knowles enjoys spending time with her grandchildren, who bring joy and pleasure into her otherwise dull life.

PODIATRIC PRESENTATION

Mrs Knowles has rigid, high-arched feet with deep-seated, painful corns over the metatarsal heads. Podiatry treatment is required every 3–4 weeks to keep her pain-free and able to walk comfortably.

Mrs Knowles has been a patient in the practice for over 3 years and has developed a friendly and comfortable relationship with the podiatrist. Over a period of 2–3 months the podiatrist notices that Mrs Knowles is becoming distant and appears very tired. On some occasions conversation between them has become uncharacteristically stilted and the podiatrist notices that Mrs Knowles is becoming evasive. At about this time the podiatrist also notices that Mrs Knowles is using an increasing amount of perfume. As the weeks pass this becomes more obvious until the podiatrist feels obliged to comment. At this point Mrs Knowles finally breaks down and reveals that she had been very worried about her health for some months.

She says, 'Would you mind if I showed you what's been troubling me? It's got nothing to do with my feet, but I don't know who else to turn to.'

Mrs Knowles unbuttons her blouse and removes layers of bandages and padding from her breast, finally revealing what is obviously a fungating tumour. The wound is deep, with a purulent, offensive discharge. Mrs Knowles starts to cry.

She explains that she has been terrified to go to her doctor for a number of reasons. She is fearful of a diagnosis of cancer, believing that this is always fatal. She is also concerned about letting her daughter and grandchildren down, worrying that treatment might involve hospitalization. In addition, a stay in hospital would mean that her daughter could not work. Mrs Knowles fears that she will not be able to help with the grandchildren and that she would inevitably lose touch with them. She also believes that any treatment for cancer would inevitably necessitate prolonged aftercare and convalescence, which would result in her becoming a 'burden' to her daughter.

FACTORS INFLUENCING MARGARET'S BEHAVIOUR

Illness behaviour and perceptions of illness are important concepts. The same 'illness' may be experienced differently by different people and has different meanings for them. This individual experience of illness results in people behaving in individual ways (Kasl & Cobb 1966).

Furthermore, the patient's perception of symptoms may not correlate with the seriousness of the condition. Patients' perceptions of illness or disease severity often have a cultural component, and the manner in which the individual is meant to respond is then culturally determined.

People from different cultural backgrounds report pain differently and behave in different ways, which are acceptable to, and expected in, their cultures. In a seminal piece of work conducted in a New York hospital, Zborowski (1952), reported that male Jewish patients tended to articulate their feelings with 'passion'. By contrast, what Zborowski described as 'old American' (Caucasian non-Jewish) patients behaved with stoicism because emotional outbursts were viewed by their families as embarrassing. Italians and patients from Hispanic cultures, on the other hand, behaved similarly and when in pain demonstrated great emotional outbursts of sorrow and anger. Such behaviour was regarded as acceptable by Italian and Hispanic families.

A patient's perception of their illness is dependent upon their previous experience and knowledge of that condition. Symptoms do not always result in medical consultation. When people experience unusual, abnormal or persistent symptoms, they turn to what is known as the 'lay referral system'. This involves consulting family and friends for advice about their condition (Cameron et al 1995). More importantly, it is through the lay referral system that the patient learns how s/he is *meant to respond* to the symptoms in a way that is normatively acceptable.

Seeking professional help may be further delayed as a result of fear, ignorance of the condition and embarrassment. The way in which patients describe their symptoms varies widely and is also affected by cultural and demographic factors. Many people who experience symptoms choose to wait to see whether they develop further before seeking professional advice.

Disease is not always characterized by the presence of symptoms. Even when symptoms are present, the pattern of their presentation is not always consistent. The lay referral system also serves to interpret what may be confusing and unfamiliar experiences. Leventhal & Binyamini (1997) suggest that the relationship between symptoms and diagnosis is in some ways reciprocal: people who experience symptoms tend to seek a diagnosis while people who are given a diagnosis tend to seek symptoms consistent with it.

Not all people respond to symptoms in ways that appear logical. Reactions to symptoms and lay beliefs about illness may result in behaviours that can range from complete denial of the illness through to a preoccupation with somatic symptoms. It is the task of the podiatrist to tease out a patient's health beliefs in order to reach an understanding of their illness perceptions. An understanding of the patient's perspective, and thus behaviour, enables the podiatrist to tailor support to meet their needs.

Various models have been proposed to explain illness behaviour. Kasl & Cobb (1966) proposed a structuralist approach (Fig. 13.1). This suggests that people's behaviour, attitudes and values occur as a result of the organization and structure of the society in which they live. The approach does not explain why people with similar social characteristics behave differently on experiencing similar symptoms.

As long ago as 1956, Beecher noted that individuals with injuries resulting in similar physical damage reacted differently. The manner in which the injury occurred determined the way in which the resultant damage was perceived. Injuries sustained by soldiers that resulted in the granting of home leave were evaluated differently from similar injuries suffered by factory workers in their work place. Beecher (1956) suggests that for the soldiers

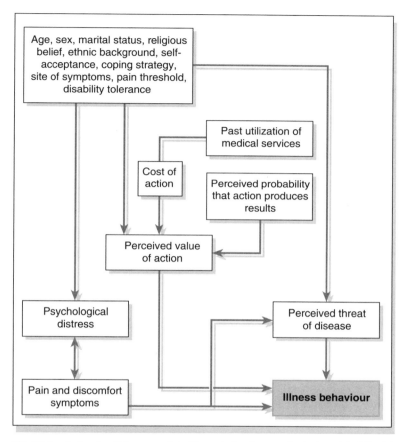

Fig. 13.1   A structuralist approach to illness behaviour – adapted model of Kasl & Cobb (1966) from Bond & Bond (1994)

the benefits resulting from the injury might compensate for the costs involved. In addition, soldiers injured during active service requested fewer doses of analgesia than did civilians injured in the work place who suffered comparable injuries. This might explain why Margaret has been reluctant to seek advice regarding her breast tumour. Her need to continue to assist her daughter and grandchildren is greater than her need to seek help for her medical condition. The apparent illogicality of Margaret's behaviour is thus in reality easily understood.

When patients become ill they seek ways to explain and understand what has happened to them. It may be hard to make sense of what has happened, particularly if they have never experienced the symptoms or have merely been given a diagnosis. People often ask 'Why me?' 'Why now?', seeking explanations for their predicament based on considerations of personal history, lifestyle and behaviour.

For some people, their symptoms must be taken seriously by *others* before the sufferer regards them as legitimate and can therefore define themselves as being ill (Senior & Viveash 1998). People develop theories about their illness through consideration of their own experience and that of their families and friends, and from knowledge gained from the media. Scharloo et al (1998) suggests that there are five dimensions to the perceptions of illness:

* The problem, including signs, symptoms and labelling
* The cause of the problem
* The consequences of the problem
* The natural history and prognosis of the illness
* The cure/controllability of the illness.

Some or all of these dimensions are considered by the individual when making decisions about their health behaviour.

Heider (1958) proposed explanations for how people view their own behaviour and that of others. These explanations have become known as attribution theory. Attribution is said to be operationalized in two different ways. The first is known as dispositional attribution, in which a person's behaviour may be explained by the presence of a stable characteristic, for example always being late. The second is known as situational attribution in which a behaviour may be explained by external factors over which the individual has no personal control, for example being late as a result of traffic congestion.

In Mrs Knowles's case it may be that dispositional and situational attributions have combined to prevent her from seeking advice for her condition. On one hand Mrs Knowles's disposition is such that she stoically refuses to 'make a fuss' about her own health. On the other hand she has a daughter who is a lone parent and needs her help. Together these factors may explain her behaviour.

In general, people's health status is influenced by their social, environmental and economic circumstances in addition to their access to and uptake of medical services. People in higher socio-economic groups enjoy better health and enjoy lower morbidity and mortality rates than do those in lower socioeconomic groups (Phillimore et al 1994).

Challenge 1: How can you deal with Margaret's distress in a way that is helpful to her?

When patients express powerful emotions such as sadness, grief and anxiety it may be difficult for you not to share these feelings with your patients. If you lack the skills to deal with your patients' emotions appropriately, you may feel inadequate and uncomfortable. Margaret's situation is such that it is unlikely that anyone would be prepared adequately for the emotional impact her case presents.

When a person is acutely upset it is important not to attempt to prevent them from expressing emotion. It is helpful to find a private space away from others so that their distress is not further compounded by embarrassment.

When the patient has regained some composure, they should be allowed to articulate their concerns without pressure or interruption. Most importantly, the podiatrist should listen to what their patient is saying. Specialist counselling skills and qualifications are not required to be of real help and comfort to people who are acutely distressed. A warm and empathetic response and an expression of concern can be very effective in ameliorating such situations. After the patient has left the clinic it is important for the podiatrist to reflect on how s/he has handled the situation and how s/he might respond better in future. This process is often referred to as reflective practice.

Reflective practice is a primary skill based on self-awareness. It links what we know, feel and think to what we observe in our selves and in others. This process helps to formalize how the practitioner views the world, and how s/he organizes and interprets information in professional practice. Where there is misunderstanding between the patient and the podiatrist, conflict and feelings of unease can occur. Reflective practice allows the podiatrist to learn from experience and to prevent the occurrence of similar problems in the future. It is thus very important for podiatrists to reflect on how their reaction to patients' feelings influences their own feelings and actions.

Challenge 2: How can you moderate your own responses to unpleasant or frightening stimuli in order to avoid embarrassing your patient?

There will be times when you will be presented with sights that may be alarming and smells that are far from pleasant. In such situations it is important that you maintain a professional and non-judgemental demeanour. It may be helpful to engage in general conversation to distract the patient from any non-verbal signals that you maybe displaying inadvertently. It is also helpful to make regular eye contact and maintain a warm and friendly manner. When advice is being offered, particularly with regard to personal hygiene, a neutral and non-judgemental approach should be employed.

With experience you will find that you react less acutely to unpleasant sights and smells. You will find that you are able to tolerate such situations without displaying signs of distaste. Inevitably, this results in a better and more comfortable experience for both you and the patient.

MARGARET KNOWLES: SUMMARY OF IMPORTANT HEALTH PSYCHOLOGY

The social factors which determine Margaret Knowles's actions are more significant to her than her medical needs. It is important for podiatrists to have a clear understanding of the motivations and values of their patients in order to act in a non-discriminatory and non-judgemental way. In order to achieve such understanding, podiatrists need to have an understanding of the basis of illness behaviour.

Patients often behave in ways that may not appear logical to the podiatrist at first sight.

FURTHER READING

Bond J, Bond S 1994 Sociology and health care. An introduction for nurses and other health care professionals, 2nd edn. Churchill Livingstone, Edinburgh
Gwyn R 2001 Communicating health and illness. Sage, London
Niven N 2000 Health psychology for health care professionals, 3rd edn. Churchill Livingstone, Edinburgh
Wilkinson RG 1997 Unhealthy societies: the afflictions of inequality. Routledge, London

REFERENCES

Beecher HK 1956 Relationship of significance of wound to pain experienced. Journal of the American Medical Association 161, 1609–1613
Bond J, Bond S 1994 Sociology and health care. An introduction for nurses and other health care professionals, 2nd edn. Churchill Livingstone, Edinburgh
Cameron L, Leventhal EA, Leventhal H 1995 Seeking medical care in response to symptoms and life stress. Psychosomatic Medicine 57, 37–47
Heider F 1958 The psychology of interpersonal relations. John Wiley, New York
Kasl SA, Cobb S 1966 Health behaviour and illness behaviour and sick role behaviour. Archives of Environmental Health 12, 246–266
Leventhal H, Binyamini Y 1997 Lay beliefs about health and illness. In Baum A, Newman S, Weinman J et al (ed) Cambridge handbook of psychology, health and medicine. Cambridge University Press, Cambridge, pp. 72–77
Phillimore P, Beattie A, Townsend P 1994 The widening gap. Inequality of health in northern England 1981–1991. British Medical Journal 308, 1125–1128
Scharloo M, Kapstein AA, Weinman J et al 1998 Illness perceptions: coping and functioning in patients with rheumatoid arthritis, chronic obstructive pulmonary disease and psoriasis. Journal of Psychosomatic Medicine 44, 573–585
Senior M, Viveash B 1998 Health and illness. Macmillan, London
Zborowski M 1952 Cultural components in response to pain. Journal of Social Issues 8, 16–30

14

Dorothy Atkins – the importance of self-efficacy

From quiet homes and first beginning,
Out to the undiscovered ends,
There's nothing worth the wear of winning,
But laughter and the love of friends.

Hilaire Belloc

Dorothy is a 63-year-old married woman who has two grown-up children and four 'delightful' grandchildren. Dorothy and her husband have had a very happy life and have enjoyed her husband's retirement. They have lots of friends, have an active social life, being members of the local bowls club and horticultural society, and enjoy spending time with their family. Dorothy is a very happy person and feels that she has had a fulfilled and satisfying life.

Six months ago, Dorothy detected a small lump in her right breast, which was diagnosed as cancerous and has resulted in Dorothy having a mastectomy and a course of chemotherapy. Dorothy has been very optimistic throughout this period and believes that the treatment will return her to full health. She has been supported by her family and friends and has also joined the local support group, which she has found most beneficial.

PODIATRIC PRESENTATION

Dorothy has attended the podiatrist recently for treatment of a fungal infection.

FACTORS INFLUENCING DOROTHY'S BEHAVIOUR

Dorothy is a very positive, optimistic person who has derived much of strength from her supportive family and from her network of friends.

IMPORTANT PSYCHOLOGICAL THEORY

Dorothy exhibits optimism and a high degree of self-efficacy. Self-efficacy is a characteristic that represents the degree of confidence a person has in their ability to perform certain behaviours. Self-efficacy has been shown to be associated with a variety of health outcomes (Grembowski et al 1993). Optimism is regarded as displaying favourable expectations for the future.

There is evidence to suggest that social support and ongoing membership of a social network are important in maintaining self-efficacy in later life. McAvay et al (1996) found that a decline in health and self-efficacy was related to poorer social networks and fewer social contacts. There is also evidence of the reciprocal nature of the relationship between self-efficacy and social support: the impact of social support is to enhance self-efficacy, and vice versa (Holahan & Holahan 1987).

Dorothy also demonstrates a high degree of hardiness, which is related to self-efficacy and is characterized by a sense of personal control and commitment. Hardiness provides Dorothy with some of the emotional strength that helps her deal with her condition. She also holds very strong beliefs about the causes and consequences of her illness. These beliefs have been developed through her wide reading about cancer and cancer treatments.

Dorothy also believes strongly that she can influence the outcome of her illness. She also shows a strong general motivation, a characteristic necessary to obtain positive outcomes (Dunn 1996).

Locus of control is a concept that has been applied very widely in health psychology. The original theory was proposed by Rotter (1966) and has been the subject of much psychological research. People are said to have an *internal locus of control* if they believe that they have the ability to control events around them. By contrast, people are said to have an *external locus of control* if they believe that things that happen to them are largely controlled by outside influences.

Levenson (1981) later suggested that the concept of locus of control was multidimensional. He proposed that external control had two components: the belief that events are random and controlled by chance and the belief that events are under the control of powerful others. Other authors have applied the concept to health-related behaviours. Wallston and coworkers (Wallston & Wallston 1978, Wallston et al 1994) developed the original health locus of control scale, which is composed of internal locus of control (IHLC), powerful others locus of control (PHLC), and chance locus of control (CHLC). Although medical practitioners were the subject of the 'powerful others' dimension in Wallston's original work, it has been recognized more recently that a wider range of individuals may be substantially influential on an individual's behaviour.

It is important for the podiatrist to assess Dorothy's health knowledge and explore her health beliefs because these can be influential. This concept is explored in detail in the character of *James Watt* in Chapter 6. When in discussion with patients, it is important for practitioners to recognize that patients have access to a wide range of health-related information that will significantly influence their behavioural beliefs. It is also very important to be aware that a patient's friends and family play a pivotal role in their recovery.

Challenge 1: Explain why Dorothy is able to remain so cheerful despite having been diagnosed with a life-threatening condition

Many studies have demonstrated the independent effect of social networks on health status, morbidity and mortality rates. Perhaps the most important of these studies was conducted in Alameda County, California (Seeman et al 1987). Nearly 7000 adults were studied over a 9-year period. At the beginning of the period, subjects' social networks were recorded. Notes were taken of subjects' number of relatives, friends, membership of church and social groups and of the contact that the subject had with supportive others. Mortality and morbidity rates were then recorded in the same cohort 9 years later. The study demonstrated clearly that those people with poorer social and community ties were far more likely to have died during the study period than those who had better social networks. The age-adjusted relative risks for socially isolated people compared to those with the most social contacts were 2.3 for men and 2.8 for women. This effect was found to be independent of self-reported physical health status at the beginning of the study, year of death, socioeconomic status and all major health behaviours such as cigarette smoking, alcohol consumption, obesity, physical inactivity and use of health services. Similar findings have been reported in a prospective study of elderly men in Sweden (Hanson et al 1990). Five hundred men born in 1914 were interviewed and examined in 1982/3. A higher mortality risk was found for men with a lower availability of emotional support and those who reported lower levels of social participation. This was particularly the case for men who lived alone. In these subjects, the relative risks for mortality were found to be in the range of 2.2–2.5 after adjustments had been made for social class, health status at baseline, cardiovascular risk factors, alcohol intake, physical activity and body mass index.

More recently, an 11-year longitudinal study of elderly men and women in Denmark showed a similar independent association between social relations and mortality risks. In this study social relations were assessed by:

- Structural considerations such as household composition, the presence of children and contact of frequency with relatives
- The function of social relations such as support with activities of daily living
- Participation in tasks that bring individuals together, such as volunteer work.

The study not only showed an association between social relations and mortality consistent with the American and Swedish studies but also demonstrated that two aspects of social relationships were particularly important. Firstly, it is important for individuals to receive support with a range of everyday tasks. Secondly it appears to be protective to help others, thus providing a sense of belonging and of usefulness to society.

In addition to improving quality of life and longevity, there is evidence to show that strong social networks may prevent or reduce disease processes, particularly in middle-aged and older people. A very large study ($n > 32\,000$) of male health professionals in the USA aged 42–77 entered the study in 1988 (Kawachai et al 1997). At the time, all participants were free from known coronary heart disease, stroke and cancer. Four years later, a total of 511 of the subjects had died. Socially isolated men (defined as unmarried, with fewer than six friends or relatives and with no membership of church or community groups) were found to be at increased risk of cardiovascular disease, accidents and suicide. Socially isolated men were also found to have an increased risk of stroke of more than twice that of men with the most extensive social networks. While the study found no evidence for the effects of social networking on non-fatal heart disease, it concluded that social networks assist in prolonging the survival of men with established cardiovascular disease.

Many articles have supported the findings of the studies reported above. More recently Lisa Berkman (Berkman et al 2000), one of the authors of the seminal work in this field, has suggested mechanisms by which social networks may influence individual health status. Berkman's explanations are drawn from a wide range of theory ranging from sociology to psychoanalysis. An important strand of Berkman's explanation is based on attachment theory (Bowlby 1969). Bowlby argued that the separation of infants from mothers represented an unhealthy loss, resulting in a universal human need to form close, affectionate bonds. According to attachment theory, the attached figure, generally the mother, creates a secure base from which the developing child can explore. Bowlby developed this proposal to the extent of suggesting that 'secure attachment provides an external ring of psychological protection which maintains the child's metabolism in a stable state similar to internal homeostatic mechanisms of blood pressure and temperature control'. It is these attachments formed in infancy that are said to provide a basis for attachment in adulthood. Individuals whose attachment in infancy is ambivalent or disorganized may be less able to form secure attachment in adulthood.

Fifty years ago anthropologists developed the concept of social networks to describe relationships that were independent of traditional family residential and social class groups. Analysis of social networks was concerned with understanding the patterns of ties between actors in a social system rather than on characteristics of the individuals themselves (Hall & Wellman 1985). Thus individual behaviour is largely determined by the social structure of the network rather than individual differences of its members. Berkman identifies a range of characteristics of social networks that are particularly influential:

- The range or number of network members
- The extent to which the members are connected to each other
- The degree to which they are defined on the basis of traditional structures, e.g. family, work or neighbourhood
- The extent to which individuals are similar within a network.

The characteristics of individual ties within the network include:

- Frequency of contact
- The number of types of transactions of support provided by a set of ties
- The length of time one individual knows another
- The extent to which exchanges are reciprocated.

Berkman postulates that social isolation, disintegration and disconnectedness influence mortality by influencing the rate of ageing. She hypothesizes that social isolation is 'a chronically stressful condition to which the organism responded by ageing faster ... the cumulative conditions which tend to occur in very old age [are] accelerated'.

There is biological support for this hypothesis. Rats that are handled frequently and early in life have been shown to recover faster from the effects of stressful stimuli than rats that have never been handled or that are experiencing maternal separation. Moreover, rats that were not handled showed age-related rises in hormones that were not found among rats that had experienced early handling.

It is very clear from the evidence currently available that direct pathways exist between people's social lives, personal interactions and sense of belonging and their biologically defined state of health or illness. This effect is extraordinarily powerful and should never be underestimated as an important determinant of patients' general state of health.

Challenge 2: How do you refuse gifts without causing offence?

Dorothy takes pleasure in bringing a small gift to the podiatrist each time she comes for an appointment. Recently the employing authority has issued a policy stating that 'gifts from patients should not be accepted'. How do you deal with this without causing offence?

DOROTHY ATKINS: SUMMARY OF IMPORTANT HEALTH PSYCHOLOGY

The important psychological issues to be considered in the case of Dorothy Atkins are her positive traits and also the positive effect of her strong family and social ties. Patients like Dorothy do not present an personal challenge in practice and fortunately are in the majority.

FUTHER READING

Kaplan G 1996 People and places; contrasting perspectives on the association between social class and health. International Journal of Health Services 26, 507–519

Marmot M, Wilkinson RG 1999 Social determinants of health. Oxford University Press, Oxford

Wilkinson RG 1997 Unhealthy societies: the afflictions of inequality, 2nd edn. Routledge, London

REFERENCES

Berkman L, Glass T, Brissette Seeman TE 2000 From social integration to health: Durkheim in the new millennium. Social Science and Medicine 51, 543–857

Bowlby J 1969 Attachment and loss. Hogarth Press, London

Dunn DS 1996 Well being following amputation: salutary effects of positive meaning, optimism and control. Rehabilitation Psychology 41, 285–302

Grembowski D, Patrick D, Diehr P et al 1993 Self efficacy and health behaviour among older adults. Journal of Health and Social Behavior 34, 89–104

Hall A, Wellman B 1985 Social networks and social support. In Cohen S, Syme SL (ed) Social support and health. Academic Press, Orlando, FL, p. 23–41

Hanson BS, Isacsson SO, Janzon L, Lindell SE 1990 Social support and quitting smoking for good: is there an association? Results from the population study 'Men born in 1914', Malmo, Sweden. Addictive Behaviors 15, 221–233

Holahan C, Holahan C 1987 Self-efficacy, social support and depression in aging: a longitudinal analysis. Journal of Gerontology 42, 65–68

Kawachai I, Kennedy BP, Lochner K, Prowthrow-Stith D 1997 Social capital, income inequality, and mortality. American Journal of Public Health 87, 1491–1498

Levenson H 1981 Differentiating among internality, powerful others and chance. In Lefcourt HM (ed) Research with the locus of control construct, vol 1. Academic Press, New York

McAvay GJ, Seeman TE, Rodin J 1996 A longitudinal study of change in domain-specific self efficacy among older adults. Journals of Gerontology Series B, Psychological Sciences and Social Sciences 51, 243–253

Rotter JB 1966 Generalised expectancies for the internal versus external control of reinforcement theory. Psychological Monographs 901, 1–28

Seeman TE, Kaplan GA, Knudsen L et al 1987 Social network ties and mortality among the elderly in the Alameda County Study. American Journal of Epidemiology 126, 714–723

Wallston KA, Wallston BS 1978 Development of the multidimensional health locus of control (MHLC.) Health Education Monographs 6, 160–170

Wallston KA, Stein MJ, Smith CA 1994 Form C of the Multidimensional Health Locus of Control Scale. Journal of Personality Assessment 63, 534–553

15

Sophie Miller – a disabled adolescent with an interest in complementary medicine

Life is what happens while you are making other plans.

John Lennon

Sophie is a slightly overweight 17-year-old girl who was born with spina bifida. She is unable to walk unaided and spends much of her time in a wheelchair. She is a bright and lively girl who lives at home with her parents and her little brother, who is 7 years old. Sophie has aspirations to have a career in business administration, and when she left school at 16 she started at the local technical college, where she enrolled in a secretarial course. Unfortunately, her health was not good during her first year at college, which resulted in a lot of time absent from her studies. She has had to intermit from the course but hopes to restart it at the beginning of the next academic year.

Her parents are unemployed and live on benefits, and they find looking after Sophie difficult and a full-time job. Her father has tried to find work but is not committed to finding a job because he thinks he would only be slightly better off financially.

PODIATRIC PRESENTATION

Sophie has peripheral neuropathy and has recently developed ulcers on her toes where her shoes have been rubbing. She is eligible for podiatry treatment but has a history of failing to attend for her appointments. Continuity of treatment is important for Sophie to treat her podiatric problems as and when they arise, and also to monitor her condition. Maintenance of health is of utmost importance to enable her to be independent and achieve her goals and aspirations.

The podiatry clinic sends appointments through the post and leaves phone messages on Sophie's parents' answering machine. Sophie's father refuses to use the answering machine and will not listen to any messages that are left. He does not like opening 'official-looking envelopes' because he finds them intimidating. Sophie's mother runs an open house for all the local children, welcomes them in, befriends them all and enjoys dealing with their personal problems. She is slightly embarrassed about Sophie and finds it difficult having a daughter who is handicapped.

Sophie has recently been feeling disillusioned and 'let down' by allopathic (conventional) medicine and has developed an interest in complementary and homeopathic approaches. She is keen to know whether homeopathic preparations or complementary treatments would improve her health.

FACTORS THAT INFLUENCE SOPHIE'S BEHAVIOUR

Spina bifida is a congenital deformity that usually begins between the fourth and sixth weeks of pregnancy. It is characterized by a defective closure in the vertebral column, of varying severity. There are two primary types:

• **Spina bifida occulta** is the milder form, in which the defective closure is beneath a layer of skin. It occurs when one or more of the vertebrae of the spine fail to fuse properly. There are generally no associated functional limitations.

• **Spina bifida manifesta** has two common forms. In the rare but milder form, a skin-filled sac containing cerebrospinal fluid and nerve roots appears in the lower back. The more common, severer form is characterized by a failure of the spinal cord to form a tube. A portion of the undeveloped cord protrudes through the back. The cord has a sac around it containing cerebrospinal fluid, which may be covered by skin or simply by tissue and exposed nerves.

Ultimately, the severity of spina bifida is determined by the site of the protrusion and by the nerves that are affected. Damage and symptoms occur when the spinal cord develops and the sac grows, damaging the surrounding nerves. Parts of the body corresponding to these damaged or undeveloped nerves will be impaired; there is a direct correlation between the area of the lesion and the associated paralysis or other impairment.

Disabilities or functional limitations associated with spina bifida depend upon the location of the lesion and associated nerve damage. The most common impairment is partial or total paralysis of affected muscle groups. Since most lesions are found in the low thoracic, lumbar or sacral regions of the spine, the lower extremities and bowel, bladder and sexual functions are most often involved. Ambulation must often be supplemented by wheelchairs and related aids. In more severe cases, the trunk and upper extremities are involved, further limiting independence in vocational and daily-care skills.

In 1980 the World Health Organization attempted to standardize the classification of disability internationally, and suggested that 'impairment' referred to physical or cognitive limitations that an individual might have, such as the inability to walk or speak. By contrast, 'disability' relates to socially imposed restrictions, in other words the system of social constraints that are imposed on those with impairments by the discriminatory practices of society. A handicap is a disadvantage resulting from impairment or a disability that limits or prevents the fulfilment of a role that is normal (depending on age, sex and social and cultural factors) for that individual.

Disabled people, while not necessarily ill, may encounter a variety of social disadvantages as the result of stigma (Susman 1994, Reynolds-Whyte & Ingstad 1995), which makes a person seen as different from others and thus less desirable (Breakey 1997).

Body image is concerned with the way in which an individual perceives their own body and is predicated on an internal 'model' of body shape and size (Fisher 1973). This internal model is subjective rather than objective and may be altered by psychological states.

Western society has long been preoccupied with what it considers to be the perfect human form, although the exact nature of this form has changed across history. Whatever the contemporary fashion for body shape, deviation from it is generally viewed as undesirable (Breakey 1997).

Despite her physical state, Sophie has great confidence in her own ability to succeed in her chosen career. The belief that one is able to achieve goals is often described as self-efficacy.

Self-efficacy was first described by Bandura in 1977, and is recognized as an important factor that may influence a wide range of health-related behaviours. To possess self-efficacy requires belief in one's own competence; Sophie's self-efficacy in relation to her college work and career is strong and it is very important that the podiatrist maximizes the opportunity for Sophie to draw on this strength.

In addition, Sophie is optimistic by nature and tends to latch on to any opportunity that she sees as having potential. This sometimes results in her accepting ideas uncritically and she might be regarded as slightly impressionable.

Sophie's parents provide such support as they are able. The way in which Sophie receives social support may be viewed in two ways: the support she feels she has (*perceived social support*) and the support that she actually or potentially has (*structural social support*). In reality, perceived support is often more important than simply having structures in place for support to be given (Schaefer et al 1981).

Sophie does not feel particularly well supported by her parents. She considers herself to be more intelligent and better motivated than her father and resents the attention her mother gives to the other local children. Sophie is thus particularly vulnerable to the social influence of other people who are important in her life, notably her teachers, college friends and the range of health professionals involved in her care. Sophie's self-efficacy, independence and optimism combine to make her on the one hand keen to maximize her potential through hard work but on the other hand difficult to persuade to engage with her treatment unless she is thoroughly convinced of its efficacy.

Sophie has recently visited a complementary medicine centre and feels that the treatment she received there was more beneficial than her conventional treatment. Sophie is particularly interested in homeopathy and has consulted a practitioner regarding her ulcerated toes. There is limited evidence concerning the efficacy of homeopathic medicine in podiatry, although homeopathic remedies have been investigated as alternative to some conventional podiatric treatments (Concha et al 1998, Khan & Khan 2000a, b). However, Sophie is worried that the podiatrist may be dismissive of all complementary therapies because she perceives the podiatrist as part of the 'medical establishment'.

Homeopathy, or homeopathic medicine, is a system of treatment that originated in the late 18th century. The name homeopathy is derived from two Greek words that mean 'like' and 'disease'. Homeopathy is based on the idea that substances that produce symptoms of illness in healthy people will have a curative effect when given in very dilute quantities to sick people who exhibit the same symptoms.

Homeopathic remedies are believed to stimulate the body's own healing processes. Samuel Hahnemann (1755–1843), the founder of homeopathic medicine, used the Latin phrase *similia similibus curantur*, 'let like be cured with like', to summarize the underlying principle of his system. By contrast, homeopaths use the term 'allopathy', or 'different from disease', to describe the use of drugs in conventional medicine to oppose or counteract the symptom being treated.

The aim of homeopathy is the restoration of the body to homeostasis, or healthy balance, which is considered its natural state. The symptoms of a disease are regarded as the body's own defensive attempt to correct its imbalance, rather than as enemies to be defeated. Because a homeopath regards symptoms as positive evidence of the body's 'inner intelligence', s/he will prescribe a remedy designed to stimulate this internal curative process rather than suppress it.

Evidence-based practice dominates academic thinking and clinical medicine and has resulted in an increased emphasis on research findings and improved dissemination. However, within the past decade there has been a small but discernible move among healthcare professionals to refer patients to, and to practise, complementary therapies for the efficacy of which there is little scientific evidence (Paterson & Britten 1999).

Complementary medicine is clearly enjoying a popularity unanticipated 30 years ago. The past three decades have witnessed a rapid growth in popularity, both among conventional practitioners and among patients seeking treatment. An explanation of why these changes might have occurred is clearly of great interest to all professions based on notions of evidence-based care (Paterson & Britten 1999).

A number of studies have attempted to address this issue by exploring the reasons patients give for seeking complementary treatments. In general practice, patients report the failure of conventional medicine to help their condition as their main motivation (Vincent & Furnham 1997, Moore et al 1985). In addition, some patients use complementary medicine to supplement orthodox medicine rather than to replace it (Thomas et al 1991, Fulder & Munro 1985). More recent work identifies five key factors that help to explain this change in thinking. These are:

- A positive evaluation of complementary treatment
- The ineffectiveness of orthodox medicine
- Concerns about adverse effects of orthodox medicine
- Poor communication skills among doctors
- Concerns about the availability of complementary medicine (Vincent & Furnham 1997).

Challenge 1: How should the podiatrist view Sophie's wish to use homeopathic remedies for her ulcers?

A criticism widely applied to many complementary therapies is that their effect is entirely due to suggestion. This is generally known as a *placebo effect*. A placebo (Latin for 'I shall please') is any treatment that contains no known active ingredient. Yet a placebo often causes a measurable, observable or felt improvement in health that is reported by the patient. The reasons why an inert substance should have a therapeutic effect is unknown.

However, there is a very large body of literature that shows that placebos can be at least as effective as many active treatments.

Some researchers believe the placebo effect is entirely psychological, due to a belief in the treatment resulting in a subjective feeling of improvement. Kirsch & Sapirstein, in a controversial paper, suggested that the effectiveness of some antidepressant drugs might be attributed almost entirely to a placebo effect. They analysed 19 clinical trials of antidepressants and concluded that the expectation of improvement, not adjustments in brain chemistry, accounted for 75% of the drugs' effectiveness (Kirsch & Sapirstein 1998).

However, a person's beliefs and hopes about a treatment may have a significant biochemical effect. Both a sensory experience and thoughts can affect neurochemistry. The body's neurochemical system affects and is affected by other biochemical systems, including the hormonal and immune systems. Thus it is consistent with current knowledge that a person's hopeful attitude and beliefs may be very influential in their physical wellbeing and recovery from injury or illness.

It is also possible that at least part of the placebo effect reflects an illness or injury taking its natural course to recovery. Because of the aggressive way in which many minor conditions are now treated, the natural history of many ailments is unclear. It is thus possible that a condition that appears to respond to a placebo might have resolved itself without treatment in any case. Moreover, many disorders, pains and illnesses wax and wane. What is observed as a placebo effect may, in many cases, represent a natural regression to the mean.

However, none of these proposals is adequate to fully explain the magnitude and ubiquitousness of the placebo effect and this remains a particularly interesting area for active research.

Perhaps most importantly, much of what has been labelled a placebo effect may occur as a result of the way in which therapy is given – the process of administering therapy (Roberts et al 1993). Many consider the touching, the caring, the attention and other interpersonal communication, along with the hopefulness and encouragement provided by the therapist, to be key factors that alter the mood of the patient. This in turn triggers physical changes such as release of endorphins, which reduce stress. This reduction in stress prevents further harmful physical changes from occurring or slows them down. The process-of-treatment hypothesis may explain how the therapies offered by many complementary practitioners are often effective. It may also explain the efficacy of treatments initially thought to work by a given mechanism that is subsequently disproved.

Whether Sophie continues with her homeopathy is not an issue for the podiatrist. More important is that she continues to be monitored and provided with evidence-based podiatric treatment.

Challenge 2: How would you convince Sophie of the necessity to keep her podiatry appointments?

The most important factor in achieving this aim lies in the relationship that the podiatrist develops with Sophie. The podiatrist must respect Sophie's views about her chosen therapy. Respect is not the mere tolerance of a different viewpoint: respect requires recognition of equality between the values of the professional and those of the patient. It is this equality that is critical in maintaining Sophie's willingness to continue both in the relationship with the podiatrist and with treatment.

SOPHIE MILLER: SUMMARY OF IMPORTANT HEALTH PSYCHOLOGY

Adolescence is a time of significant physical and psychological change and development, and the exploration of the self. It is a crucial stage in the development of self-esteem and social identity. An understanding of these processes and the importance of social support in adolescence will enable the podiatrist to build an effective therapeutic relationship with Sophie. In order to do this, the podiatrist must recognize that, although Sophie's views may differ from his/her own they are no less valid and should be treated with appropriate respect.

FURTHER READING

Durkin K 1995 Developmental social psychology: from infancy to old age. Blackwell, Oxford

Fisher S, Greenberg RP 1997 From placebo to panacea: putting psychiatric drugs to the test. John Wiley, New York

Krementz J 1992 How it feels to live with a physical disability. Simon & Schuster, New York

REFERENCES

Bandura A 1977 Self efficacy. Towards a unifying theory of behavioural change. Psychological Revue 84, 191–215

Breakey JW 1997 Body image: the inner mirror. Journal of Prosthetics and Orthotics 9, 107–112

Concha JM, Steele Moore L, Holloway WJ 1998 Antifungal activity of *Melaleuca alternifolia* (tea tree oil) against various pathogenic organisms. Journal of the American Podiatry Association 88, 489–492

Fisher S 1973 Body consciousness. Open Forum, London

Fulder S, Munro R 1985 Complementary medicine in the United Kingdom. Patients, practitioners and consultants. Lancet 2, 542–545

Khan MT, Khan MT 2000a Clinical evaluation of homeopathic podiatry in the treatment of diabetic foot ulcers. British Homoeopathic Journal 89(suppl 1), S67

Khan MT, Khan MT 2000b Clinical application of homeopathic podiatry as used at The Royal London Homeopathic Hospital (RLHH). British Homoeopathic Journal 89(suppl 1), S53

Kirsch I, Sapirstein G 1998 Listening to Prozac but hearing placebo. A meta-analysis of antidepressant medication prevention and treatment. Prevention and Treatment 1, article 2a

Moore J, Phipps K, Marcer D, Lewith G 1985 Why do people seek treatment by alternative medicine? British Medical Journal 290, 28–29

Paterson C, Britten N 1999 'Doctors can't help much': the search for an alternative. British Journal of General Practice 49, 626–629

Reynolds-Whyte S, Ingstad B 1995 Disability and culture: an overview. In Ingstad B, Reynolds-Whyte S (ed) Disability and culture. University of California Press, Berkeley, CA

Roberts AH, Kewman DG, Mercier L, Hovell M 1993 The power of nonspecific effects in healing: implications for psychosocial and biological treatments. Clinical Psychology Review 13, 375–391

Schaefer C, Coyne JC, Lazarus RS 1981 The health related functions of social support. Journal of Behavioural Medicine 4, 381–406

Susman J 1994 Disability stigma and deviance. Social Science and Medicine 38, 15–22

Thomas K, Carr J, Westlake L, Williams B 1991 Use of non-orthodox and conventional healthcare in Great Britain. British Medical Journal 302, 207–210

Vincent C, Furnham A 1997 The perceived efficacy of complementary and orthodox medicine: a replication. Complementary Therapies in Medicine 5, 85–89

World Health Organization 1980 The international classification of impairments, disabilities, and handicaps. WHO, Geneva

16

George Archer – a person with diabetes who smokes

It is not I who become addicted, it is my body.

Jean Cocteau

George is a 60-year-old builder who is currently working in his own business but is looking forward to retiring shortly. He has worked continuously since he started his apprenticeship when he was 15 years old, and he is very proud of his achievements. His business is well respected throughout the local community and he is perceived by his friends and colleagues as a very honest and straightforward individual. He has two grown-up sons and three small grandchildren of whom he is very proud.

George has been an insulin-dependent diabetic for 45 years and his diabetes is well controlled. He eats a sensible diet and drinks alcohol in moderation. George has smoked cigarettes since he was a teenager. He used to smoke heavily but has recently cut down to around 15 cigarettes a day. He suffers from early peripheral vascular disease and has a mild degree of lower limb neuropathy. He has been attending the podiatry clinic for 6 months for routine care and monitoring. Continued use of tobacco is strongly associated with the development of peripheral vascular disease, which may result in ulceration and gangrene. In order to prevent development of the negative consequences of his condition it is essential that George should stop smoking.

FACTORS INFLUENCING GEORGE'S BEHAVIOUR

George is a man who believes that hard work results in a good quality of life. His status and position are important to him and he enjoys the respect that he receives from his friends and colleagues.

FACTORS LEADING TO INCREASED RISK FOR SMOKING DIABETICS

The blood supply to George's feet, particularly to his toes, is compromised by his diabetes. Nicotine is a potent vasoconstrictor, which exacerbates his problem. If the blood supply to George's feet continues to be reduced in this way, it is likely that his healing ability will be impaired and ultimately his toes may become gangrenous. In addition, smoking is also associated with large-blood-vessel disease and coronary heart disease.

Coronary artery disease is the most common form of heart disease. It results from the gradual build-up of hardened deposits called plaques in the arteries supplying the heart muscle and is called atherosclerosis.

Over time the plaques, which consist of deposits of fat, cholesterol, calcium and other cellular particulates from the blood, constrict the coronary arteries, resulting in a diminished blood flow to the heart. This reduced blood flow to the heart can result in chest pain (angina) and complete blockage of an artery can lead to ischaemia of the myocardium (a heart attack).

Many people are unaware that they are developing coronary artery disease. The disease often develops slowly and in the absence of symptoms, over a period of decades. It is not uncommon for a heart attack to be the first sign that an individual has the disease.

Diseases of the heart and circulatory system (cardiovascular disease or CVD) are the main cause of death in the UK, accounting for over 250 000 deaths in 1998 (British Heart Foundation Statistics 2000). This accounts for one in three deaths in the UK.

The main forms of CVD are coronary heart disease (CHD) and stroke. About half of all deaths from CVD are from CHD and about a quarter are from stroke. CHD by itself is the most common cause of death in the UK. One in four men and one in five women die from the disease. CHD caused over 135 000 deaths in the UK in 1998.

The rate of premature death from CHD in the UK is 58% higher for male manual workers than it is for male non-manual workers. The premature death rate from CHD for female manual workers is more than twice that for female non-manual workers.

Overall the rate of death from CHD is falling across all social groups for both men and for women in the UK. However, the death rate among men is falling faster in non-manual workers than it is in manual workers. The result is that the class-related difference in death rates is widening. It is estimated that each year 5000 lives and 47 000 working years are lost in men aged 20–64 years because of social-class inequalities in CHD death rates. Just under one in three of all deaths under 65 years reflecting social class inequalities are due to CHD.

Diabetes substantially increases an individual's risk of developing CHD. Men with non-insulin-dependent (type II) diabetes have a two- to fourfold greater annual risk of CHD, and the increased risk in women with type II diabetes is even higher (three- to fivefold; Garcia et al 1974).

Around 3% of men and women in England have diabetes (Stamler et al 1993). The prevalence of diabetes increases with age: those aged 65–74 are around 10 times more likely than those aged 25–34 to have the disease. Overall, diabetes is more prevalent in men than in women (3.3% vs 2.5%), although women aged 16–24 are more likely to have diabetes than men of a similar age.

As in many countries worldwide, diabetes is increasing in the UK. Since 1991, prevalence has increased by around two-thirds among men and by a quarter among women. About two-thirds of people with diabetes die of some form of heart or blood-vessel disease.

In type I (insulin-dependent) diabetes, the beta cells of the pancreas produce little or no insulin. Insulin is a hormone that allows the sugar glucose to enter body cells. Once glucose enters a cell, it is used as fuel. With inadequate insulin, glucose builds up in the bloodstream instead of going into the cells. The body is unable to use glucose for energy, despite high levels of it in the bloodstream. This causes symptoms such as excessive thirst, increased urine output and feelings of hunger. Within 5–10 years of diagnosis, the insulin-producing cells of the pancreas are completely destroyed and no more insulin is produced.

Type I diabetes can occur at any age, but onset is usually before 30 years of age. Symptoms are usually more severe and occur more rapidly with this type of diabetes. People with this condition require insulin to live.

The exact cause of type I diabetes is not known; however, a family history of diabetes, viruses that injure the pancreas and destruction of insulin-making cells by the body's immune system may play causative roles. Risk factors for type I diabetes include immune system diseases, viral infections and a family history of diabetes.

Insulin-dependent diabetes accounts for 3% of all new cases of diabetes each year. There is one new case per 7000 children per year. The number of new cases decreases after the age of 20.

People who smoke have a risk of heart attack that is more than twice that of non-smokers. Cigarette smoking is the biggest risk factor for sudden cardiac death. Smokers who have a heart attack are also more likely to die as a result and to do so suddenly (within an hour of onset). People who smoke cigars or pipes have an increased risk of death from coronary heart disease (and possibly stroke) compared to non-smokers, but cigarette smoking carries the highest risk. Constant exposure to other people's smoke also increases the risk of heart disease, even for non-smokers. It is estimated that about 20% of deaths from CHD in men and 17% in women are due to smoking but that only 0.5% of deaths from CHD in the UK will be avoided if the government's new targets for smoking prevalence (26% by 2005 and 24% by 2010) are met (British Heart Foundation Statistics 2000).

Gangrene is the term for the death of tissue (necrosis). There are several potential causes, including interruption of the blood supply, infection with certain bacteria and damage from freezing.

Gangrene in an extremity is due to an interruption of the blood supply to that limb. If the involved tissue remains free of infection, it shrivels up and becomes dry and dark in colour (dry gangrene). If the dead tissue becomes infected, it becomes moist (wet gangrene). Antibiotics may be used to treat the infection.

IMPORTANT PSYCHOLOGICAL THEORY

Why is smoking so difficult to give up? Many thousands of studies have been written on the psychology of cigarette smoking. Nicotine is an addictive substance but psychological dependence may often be more important than chemical addiction. The process by which many people stop smoking has been the subject of much discussion.

One of the most influential theories that has been used to understand smoking behaviour is the transtheoretical or stages of change model proposed by Prochaska & DiClemente (1983). The model suggests a circular structure, as shown in Figure 16.1.

A person in the pre-contemplation phase may be described as the 'contented smoker'. At some point most smokers begin to consider giving up smoking and by so doing move into the contemplation phase. It is at this point that the benefits of not smoking are first seen to be attractive. From this phase, the would-be ex-smoker moves into a preparation stage; this stage is characterized by activities such as disposing of ashtrays and lighters, making a date to stop, etc. If this is successful, the individual shifts to the action stage and quits smoking altogether. From this stage the individual may remain abstinent or may relapse, from which

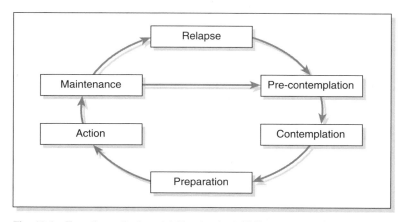

Fig. 16.1   Transtheoretical model (Prochaska & DiClemente 1983)

Table 16.1 Relative risk of death from coronary heart disease according to employment grade (from Wilkinson 1997)

Relative risk (log scale)	Class			
	Administrative	Professional/ executive	Clerical	Other
Cholesterol, smoking, other	1.0	0.3	0.9	1.4
Unexplained	0	1.8	2.3	2.6
Total	1.0	2.1	3.2	4.0

position the whole cycle may begin at a later date. Alternatively, s/he may remain permanently in the pre-contemplation stage.

It is well established that many negative health behaviours, notably smoking, a sedentary lifestyle and a high fat diet, are more common among people in lower socioeconomic groups (Table 16.1). It is therefore unsurprising to note that the prevalence of many diseases, including coronary heart disease and some cancers, follows a similar pattern.

However, it is important to understand that the socioeconomic gradient reported in both morbidity and mortality cannot be adequately explained solely in terms of differences in health-related behaviours. The work of Marmot et al (1991) involving a sample of British civil servants clearly demonstrated that traditional targets of health promotion campaigns (smoking, exercise and diet) only contribute a minor amount of variance in the observed relationship of morbidity and mortality to social class. When such variables are controlled for, the great majority of social class variation in coronary heart disease and other causes of mortality remains.

Other investigators have suggested that this variation may be due to a wide range of social factors, such as stress, poorer social support and increased risk of social isolation, which operate on psychological, neurological and immunological levels.

In George's case, it is clearly important that he should stop smoking. He is fortunate that he has a strong and supportive family network and a stable marriage. These are resources that will be invaluable assets in his attempts to give up tobacco.

Challenge 1: How could you capitalize on George's stable social environment to facilitate his attempts to stop smoking?

In order for the podiatrist to influence George's behaviour it is important for him/her to identify at which stage in the cycle George is currently situated. The aim is then to help George to move on to the next stage. For example, it would be inappropriate to discuss issues such as nicotine replacement therapy (NRT) with George if he is still in pre-contemplation, in which case it would be more helpful to encourage him to consider the benefits of stopping smoking, in terms of both his own health and the potential effect on his family. At this stage it might be helpful for George to be exposed to a cost–benefit analysis of his smoking behaviour, which could be facilitated by the podiatrist. If George is in the contemplation stage, it would be more helpful to discuss practical issues such as setting a quit date, strategies to replace smoking and NRT.

The preparation stage includes such issues as determining a date for quitting, the best circumstances for George to quit, and enrolling family and friends into helping him stop. The action stage begins when George stops smoking completely. If this stage is sustained, he moves into the 'maintenance period'. During all these stages it is important that George is encouraged and that positive reinforcement is provided. It is often useful to encourage people to substitute cigarette smoking with a more healthy activity.

Should George relapse at any stage, it is important that the podiatrist tries to help to move him on to the contemplation stage again. For many smokers, the first attempts to give up can be unsuccessful, and reinforcement and encouragement are vital to enable eventual success, but it should be noted that repeated encouragement should not become 'nagging'.

The podiatrist's ability to judge accurately George's current stage is clearly dependent upon building a successful therapeutic relationship. Therapeutic relationships are discussed in detail in Chapter 4.

Challenge 2: What other assistance can be offered to George in order to help him stop smoking?

There are many reasons why giving up smoking is difficult, but one cause is relatively straightforward to address. Among the many constituents of tobacco smoke, it is nicotine that is the most powerfully habit-forming. It is well established that most people who quit smoking successfully do so by stopping completely and suddenly as opposed to attempting to cut down before abstinence. Reducing the number of cigarettes smoked in a day is invariably accompanied by the smoker inhaling more often and more deeply so that the blood nicotine level is maintained. Smokers have been shown to be able to titrate their blood nicotine levels very accurately by this means. It is therefore very helpful if the withdrawal symptoms induced by abstinence can be alleviated. Such relief is effectively offered by any of the variety of nicotine replacement products now available over the counter. It is important that these products are used in the directed way. Nicotine is excreted from the body quite rapidly and it is important that patients do not use such preparations for excessive periods or take more than the dose recommended. It is therefore important for all health professionals to have an understanding of the NRT products on the market when offering support to smokers wishing to quit.

While the combined effect of support from a health professional and NRT can significantly improve people's chances of successfully giving up smoking, it is important to be aware that even the most effective interventions run by the most skilled professionals still have very high relapse rates. The podiatrist should not feel that his/her efforts have 'failed' if George starts smoking again. Most smokers who quit have a history of a number of relapses before they become permanently abstinent.

GEORGE ARCHER: SUMMARY OF IMPORTANT HEALTH PSYCHOLOGY

Giving up smoking is a complex and difficult process for many people. A number of models have been employed in attempts to explain how the process operates. The transtheoretical or stages of change model (Prochaska and DiClemente 1983) provides a useful framework within which the podiatrist may approach George 's smoking and provide support to help him quit.

FURTHER READING

Bond J, Bond S 1994 Sociology and health care. An introduction for nurses and other health care professionals, 2nd edn. Churchill Livingstone, Edinburgh

Helman C 2000 Culture health and illness, 4th edn. Butterworth-Heinemann, Oxford

Kozlowski LT 2001 Cigarettes, nicotine and health: a biobehavioural approach. Sage, London

Slovic P 2001 Smoking risk perception & policy. Sage, London

Wilkinson RG 1997 Unhealthy societies: the afflictions of inequality. Routledge, London

REFERENCES

British Heart Foundation Statistics 2000 Coronary heart disease statistics. British Heart Foundation statistics database annual compendium. Department of Public Health, University of Oxford, Oxford

Garcia MJ, McNamara PM, Gordon T, Kannell WB 1974 Morbidity and mortality in diabetics in the Framingham population: sixteen-year follow-up. Diabetes 23, 105–111

Marmot MG, Davey Smith G, Stansfield S et al 1991 Health inequalities among British civil servants: the Whitehall II study. Lancet 337, 1387–1393

Prochaska JO, DiClemente CC 1983 Transtheoretical therapy: toward a more integrative model of change. Psychotherapy Theory Research and Practice 19, 276–288

Stamler J, Vaccaro O, Neaton JD, Wentworth D 1993 Diabetes, other risk factors and 12 year cardiovascular mortality for men screened in the Multiple Risk Factor Intervention Trial. Diabetes Care 16, 434–444

Wilkinson RG 1997 Unhealthy societies: the afflictions of inequality. Routledge, London

Glossary

Abnormal grief: An atypical grief reaction. It may involve an absent or prolonged period, which may include feelings of guilt, sadness and anxiety.

Acceptance: Conformity that involves both acting and believing in accord with social pressure.

Addiction: Any psychological or physiological overdependence.

Aggression: An angry emotion induced by frustration or thwarting of one's own goals. Aggression induced by anger.

Altruism: A motive to increase another's welfare without conscious regard for one's self-interests.

Anger: Anger is often defined as a strong emotional response, including both a physiological and emotional reaction. It is often exhibited when goals or aspirations are blocked especially if such action is perceived as intentional or avoidable.

Assertive behaviour: Self-expressive, honest, direct, self-enhancing, not hurtful to others, partially composed of content (feelings, rights, facts, opinions, requests, limits). It is also partially composed of non-verbal style (eye contact, voice, posture, facial expression, gestures, distance, timing, fluency, listening), appropriate for the person and the situation, rather than universal. It is being socially responsible, and is a combination of learned skills. It is not an inborn trait.

Assertiveness: Behaviour that enables a person to act in his/her own best interests, to stand up for him/herself without undue anxiety, to express honest feelings comfortably or to exercise personal rights without denying the rights of others.

Attitudes: A favourable or unfavourable evaluative reaction towards something or someone, based on one's beliefs, feelings or intended behaviour.

Attribution theory: The theory of how people explain the behaviour of others, e.g. by attributing it either to internal dispositions (enduring traits, motives and attitudes) or to external situations.

Availability heuristic: An efficient but fallible rule of thumb that judges the likelihood of things in terms of their availability in memory. If instances of something come readily to mind, we presume it to be commonplace.

Beliefs: An emotional acceptance of something, a statement or a doctrine.

Bereavement: A term used to describe the characteristic responses to the loss of a loved one.

Body image: The subjective image of one's own body. Some use the term for only physical appearance, others include functions, movement or coordination. Disturbed or inappropriate body image occurs in neurotic disturbances.

Case-based learning: An educational strategy in which the learner works in a self-directed manner toward the understanding or resolution of a practice-related issue.

Catharsis: Emotional release. The catharsis view of aggression is that aggressive drive is reduced when one 'releases' aggressive energy, either by acting aggressively or by fantasizing aggression.

Cognitive dissonance: Tension that arises when one is simultaneously aware of two inconsistent cognitions. For example, dissonance may occur when we realize that we have, with little justification, acted contrary to our attitudes or made a decision favouring one alternative despite reasons favouring another.

Compliance: Conformity that involves publicly acting in accord with social pressure while privately disagreeing. Obedience is acting in accord with a direct order.

Concordance: Achieving agreement; adherence to treatment programmes.

Conflict: A perceived incompatibility of actions or goals.

Conformity: A change in behaviour or belief as a result of real or imagined group pressure.

Coping strategies: Conscious, rational ways for dealing with the anxieties of life.

Culture: The enduring behaviours, ideas, attitudes, and traditions shared by a large group of people and transmitted from one generation to the next.

Depression: A mood state characterized by a sense of inadequacy, a decrease in activity, pessimism and sadness.

Disempowerment: To feel disempowered is to feel insignificant, with a sense that your life has little meaning. You feel a lack of control over things that really matter to you personally. You feel like an outsider who is not included or asked to help. You feel that people do not appreciate you as much as you would like.

Displacement: The redirection of aggression to a target other than the source of the frustration. Generally, the new target is a safer or more socially acceptable target.

Empathy: A cognitive awareness and understanding of the emotions and feelings of another person.

Empowerment: To feel empowered is to have a sense of wellbeing and a sense that your life has important meaning.

You have a good sense of identity and some control over things that really matter to you personally. You care about others and feel that you belong and are accepted, that you are asked to help in important ways and that you are appreciated for who you are and what you can do.

Equity: A condition in which the outcomes people receive from a relationship are proportional to what they contribute to it.

Fear: An emotional state in the presence of anticipation of a noxious stimulus. It is usually characterized by an internal subjective experience of extreme agitation, a desire to flee or attack and by a range of sympathetic reactions.

Health psychology: A field of psychology primarily concerned with health-related behaviour.

Heuristic: A method for discovery, a procedure for problem solving.

Illusion of control: Perception of uncontrollable events as subject to one's control or as more controllable than they are.

Individualism: Giving priority to one's own goals over group goals and defining one's identity in terms of personal attributes rather than group identifications.

Instinctive behaviour: An innate, unlearned behaviour pattern exhibited by all members of a species.

Learned helplessness: The hopelessness and resignation learned when a human or animal perceives no control over repeated bad events.

Locus of control: The extent to which people perceive outcomes as internally controllable by their own efforts and actions or as externally controlled by chance or outside forces.

Mediation: An attempt by a neutral third party to resolve a conflict by facilitating communication and offering suggestions.

Menarche: The first menstrual period.

Menopause: The cessation of menstrual periods.

Moral exclusion: The perception of certain individuals or groups as outside the boundary within which one applies moral values and rules of fairness. Moral inclusion is regarding others as within one's circle of moral concern.

Morbidity rate: The number of cases of a disease or disorder per unit of population (usually given as per 100 000) in a given period of time (usually per year).

Mortality rate: Specifically the death rate, usually given as number of deaths per unit of population (usually per 100 000) in a specific time (usually per year).

Motivation: The psychosocial explanation considers motivation to be an internal state that drives a person into action.

Need to belong: A motivation to bond with others in relationships that provide ongoing positive interactions.

Negative reinforcement: A procedure or method of training that uses negative reinforcers.

Normative influence: Conformity based on a person's desire to fulfil others' expectations, often to gain acceptance.

Persuasion: The process by which a message induces change in beliefs, attitudes or behaviours.

Positive reinforcement: A procedure or method of training that uses positive reinforcers.

Prejudice: A negative prejudgement of a group and its individual members.

Professionalization: The term used to describe the process by which professions change and the characteristics of and reasons for this change

Representative heuristic: The tendency to presume, sometimes despite contrary odds, that someone or something belongs to a particular group if it resembles (represents) a typical member.

Role: A set of norms that define how people in a given social position ought to behave.

Role ambiguity: Occurs when there is insufficient information to perform a job well.

Role conflict: A situation where a person is expected to perform in two or more ways that conflict in fundamental ways with each other.

Role model: An ideal, a standard, an example set up as worthy of imitation or copying.

Self-awareness: A self-conscious state in which attention focuses on oneself. It makes people more sensitive to their own attitudes and dispositions.

Self-disclosure: Revealing intimate aspects of oneself to others.

Self-efficacy: A sense that one is competent and effective, distinguished from self-esteem, one's sense of self-worth.

Self-esteem: The positive feelings of self-worth that give rise to a person's overall positive self-evaluation.

Self-image: An individual's self-concept. It is both a belief in self and a respect for self. In children, self-image is formed largely by how they think significant adults in their lives perceive them.

Self-perception theory: The idea that, when we are unsure of our attitudes, we infer them much as would someone observing us, by looking at our behaviour and the circumstances under which it occurs.

Sick role: A state that occurs when a patient adopts the role of being a patient or an invalid.

Social comparison: Evaluating one's abilities and opinions by comparing oneself to others.

Social exchange theory: The theory that human interactions are transactions that aim to maximize one's rewards and minimize one's costs.

Social identity: The 'we' aspect of our self-concept. The part of our answer to 'Who am I?' that comes from our group memberships.

Social learning theory: The theory that we learn social behaviour by observing and imitating and by being rewarded and punished.

Social psychology: The scientific study of how individuals and groups interact.

Social representations: Socially shared beliefs and widely held ideas and values, including our assumptions and cultural ideologies. Our social representations help us make sense of our world.

Social responsibility norm: An expectation that people will help those dependent upon them.

Stereotype: A belief about the personal attributes of a group of people. Stereotypes are sometimes overgeneralized, inaccurate and resistant to new information.

Stress: A state of psychological tension as a result of physiological, psychological and/or social pressures.

Vulnerability: Psychological and sociological exposure resulting in injury.

Index

Page numbers in *italics* refer to figures.

A

Acquired immune deficiency
    syndrome (AIDS) 94, 95
    see also Human immunodeficiency
        virus (HIV)
Active/passive typology of
    therapeutic relationships 35
Addiction
    case studies
        Harriet Edmondson 25, 99–108
        James Watt 15, 18, 51–59
    definition 147
    eating disorder as 103
    exercise ('buzz'/'runner's high')
        52, 54, 100
    theories 44–45, 141–142
    see also Smoking
Adjustment heuristic 38
Adolescence 100–102, 106–107,
        134–135
    case studies
        Harriet Edmondson 25, 99–108
        Sophie Miller 127–136
Ageing 27, 28, 124–125
Ageism 11
Aggression
    case studies
        Suzi Dalton 14, 15, 27–40
        Margaret Knowles 18, 109–117
        James Watt 15, 18, 51–59
    definition 147
    gender differences 56
    in grief reaction 68, 69
    management 18, 32–38, 57
    theories 57
    type A personality 52
AIDS 94, 95
    see also Human immunodeficiency
        virus (HIV)

Alcohol 73, 81, 82, 137
    and diabetes 46, 48
Altruism
    definition 147
    vs professionalization 15
Amenorrhoea 104
Anchoring 38
Anger *see* Aggression
Anorexia nervosa
    case study, Harriet Edmondson 25,
        99–108
    causes and features 102–104
    management 104–105, 107
Anxiety
    client, management of 105–106
    practitioner 24–25
Asian immigrants
    case study, Sheetal Joshi 14, 61–66
    health problems 62, 63
Assertiveness
    definition 147–148
    practitioner 54
Attachment theory 123–124
Attribution theory 114–115, 148
Availability heuristic 37, 148

B

Behavioural beliefs 42–43, 44, 47
Behavioural control 106
    perceived 44
Beliefs
    behavioural 42–43, 44, 47
    definition 148
    dietary 42–43, 46–47
    normative 43, 45
    religious 61, 63, 65
    theoretical models 28–29, 38–39,
        42–45

Bereavement *see* Grief reaction
'Big Five' model of personality 53
Biopsychosocial model of illness 3
Black Report 79, 80
Board of Registration of Medical
    Auxiliaries (BRMA) 10
Body image
    definition 148
    disability and 129–130
    fitness and 52, 100
    midlife changes and 27, 28, 30, 31
Breast cancer 110–111, 113–115, 119,
    120–121

C

Cardiovascular accident (CVA)
    see Stroke
Cardiovascular disease (CVD)
    see Coronary heart disease
    (CHD)
Case-based learning 1, 148
Case-mix changes 25
Change Model 141–142, 145
Children, case study, Olivia Saunders
    85–91
Client status 11
Clinical environments 4–5
Code of ethics/practice 11, 20
Cognitive control 106
Collegiality *see* Professional support
Communication
    interprofessional 55
    through interpreters 61, 63–64, *65*
Communication skills 15, 18, 32–35,
    82
    language 33–34, 36
    see also Therapeutic relationships
Complementary medicine 130–132
    case study, Sophie Miller 127–136
    placebo effect 132–134
Concordance 36, 38, 57, 58, 149
Confidentiality 96–97, 98
    use of interpreters 64
Conflicts
    beliefs *vs* motivation 43
    ideal *vs* actual self 31
    inter- and intra-professional 13
    medical *vs* social needs, case study,
        Margaret Knowles 18, 109–117
    role 19, 20, 152

Consent, parental 106
Continuous professional development
    (CPD) 20–21, 23–26
Control
    locus of 120–121, 150
    perceived behavioural 44
    types 106
Coronary heart disease (CHD)
    138–139, 140, 142
Council for Professions
    Supplementary to Medicine
    (CPSM) 10
Cuboid subluxations 87
Culture
    definition 149
    and pain perception 111, 112
    see also Asian immigrants
CVA *see* Stroke

D

Decision control 106
Decision-making processes 37–38,
    42–43
Demographic factors 28, 112
Depression
    definition 149
    following divorce 31
    following stroke 61, 62, 63
'Deviancy training' 102
Diabetes
    case studies
        George Archer 15, 137–145
        Charles Walters 14, 15, 41–50
    definition 45–46
    long-term effects 46
        in smokers 138–140
    monitoring 14–15
    multiprofessional team 47–48
    type I 46, 139–140
    type II 46, 139
Diabetes UK 48
Diet
    beliefs 42–43, 46–47
    see also Anorexia nervosa
Disability
    case study, Sophie Miller
        127–136
    and social disadvantage 129
    WHO classification 129
Discharge from care 71–72

Disempowerment 68, 149
Divorce 27, 28, 30, 31
Duty of care 96
Dying, stages of 68–69

E

Elderly clients, case studies
   George Archer 15, 137–145
   Dorothy Atkins 119–126
   Enid Hilton 15, 67–76
   Margaret Knowles 18, 109–117
Embarrassment 64, 104, 111, 112
   avoiding 115, 116
   parental 128
Emotional expression 115
Emotional suppression 52–53
Empathy 32–33, 54, 115, 149
Empowerment 72, 149–150
Endorphin release
   exercise 54
   process of administering therapy
      133–134
Ethnicity *see* Asian immigrants;
      Culture
Evidence-based practice 26
   and complementary medicine
      131–132
Exercise
   beliefs 47
   'buzz'/'runner's high' 52, 54, 100
   encouraging 48
   excessive 51, 53–54, 55–56, 87–88,
      103
Expectations
   parents 85–86, 89
   patient *vs* practitioner 33
Eye contact 34–35, 116
   avoidance of 61, 99

F

Facial expression 34–35
Faculty of Podiatric Surgery 9
Fear
   definition 150
   in grief reaction 68, 69
   of illness/injury 80, 110–111
Feedback 86

Five Factor Theory of personality 53
Footwear 28, 29, 31–32, 35, 36, 38
   point shoes 85, 87–90

G

Gangrene 137, 140
Gender balance, of podiatry
      profession 12
Gender differences
   aggression 56
   cuboid subluxations 87
   ethnicity and mortality 63
General practitioners (GPs) 93, 97, 106
Gestures 34–35
Gifts from patients 125
Grief reaction 68–71
   case study, Enid Hilton 15, 67–76
   health effects 72–74
   prolonged 74–75
Growth periods 88
Guidance/cooperative typology of
      therapeutic relationships 35
Guilt, grief reaction 69

H

Health Belief Model 28–29, 38–39
Health inequalities
   Asian immigrants 62, 63
   socioeconomic status 79–80, 82, 83,
      115, 139, 142
Health and Lifestyle National Survey
      79
Health Professions Council (HPC) 10
Health promotion approach 90
Health psychology 2–5, 150
Heuristics
   adjustment 38
   availability 37, 148
   definition 150
   representativeness 38, 151–152
'Hierarchy of needs' 86
Homeopathic medicine 131
   see also Complementary medicine
Housing 79
Human immunodeficiency virus (HIV)
   case study, Peter Brennan 93–98
   causes and risks of infection 94

Human immunodeficiency virus
(HIV) (*contd*)
cutaneous podiatric implications 95
progression to AIDS 94, 95
psychological issues 96–97
universal precautions 95–96, 98

I

Illness
definition 3
models 2, 3
patient *vs* professional conceptions
14
see also Morbidity and mortality
rates
Illness behaviour
models 112–114
and perceptions 111–112, 114, 117
Income and health 79
Induction programmes 20–21
Information
needs 105, 106
patient access to 36
preoperative 105
written 36
Ingrowing toenails 97, 99, 100, 105
Interpreters 61, 63–64, 65
Interprofessional communication 55
Interprofessional conflicts 13
Introversion 103

L

Language 33–34, 36
Lay referral system 111, 112
Ligamentous laxity 87–88
Listening, active 35
Locus of control 120–121, 150

M

Medical model of illness 2
Medical *vs* social needs, case study,
Margaret Knowles 18, 109–117
Menopause
case study, Suzi Dalton 14, 15, 27–40
definition 151

effects 30–31
and smoking 30–31
Mentoring 20
Midlife crisis 31
Morbidity and mortality rates
coronary heart disease (CHD) 139,
140, 142
definitions 151
loss of spouse 71
social networks and 122–123
socioeconomic factors 79, 142
standardized mortality rate (SMR)
80
stroke 63, 138
Motivation 86, 89, 116–117, 120, 130
definition 151
Multiprofessional team *see* Team roles;
Team work
Mutual participation typology of
therapeutic relationships 24,
35–36

N

Newly qualified podiatrists
factors influencing 17–21
likely sources of stress 19–20
stress-reducing strategies 20–21
Nicotine replacement therapy (NRT)
143, 144
Non-judgemental approach 116–117
Non-verbal behaviour
client 99
practitioner 33, 34–35, 116
Normative beliefs 43, 45

O

OCEAN mnemonic 53
Organizational problems 19
Osteoporosis 30, 88, 104
Overuse syndrome 51, 87

P

Pain 28, 29, 31–32, 38, 51
Pain perception 54–55, 58
cultural differences 111, 112

Paperwork/administration 17–18
Paralanguage *see* Non-verbal
    behaviour
Parents
    attitudes 100, 101, 128, 130
    consent 106
    expectations 85–86, 89
Passive/active typology of therapeutic
    relationships 36
Patient autonomy 36
Peer pressure 101–102
Peripheral neuropathy 127–128
Peripheral vascular disease 137
Personality
    models/theories 52–53, 54
    problems, case study, James Watt
        15, 18, 51–59
Physical appearance
    see Body image
Placebo effect 132–134
Point (ballet) shoes 85, 87–90
Power shift in therapeutic
    relationships 36
Practitioner–patient relationships
    see Therapeutic relationships
Preoperative information 105
Private practitioners
    continuous professional
        development (CPD) 20–21,
        23–26
    professional autonomy 24–25
Private *vs* health service practice 24,
    25, 80, 81–82
Problem-based learning 1–8
Professional autonomy 12–13,
    24–25
Professional boundaries 96
Professional competence 98, 105,
    107
Professional indemnity 24
Professional status 11–12, 13, 15
Professional support (collegiality) 4–5,
    18, 20–21
Professional training 2–5, 9, 13
Professionalization
    definition 151
    sociological approaches 10–11
    vs altruism 15

Q

Questioning styles 34

R

Referral 55, 74–75
Reflective practice 115–116
Registrar General's Classification of
    Occupations 78–79
Reinforcement, positive/negative 86,
    151
Religious beliefs 61, 63, 65
Representativeness heuristic 38,
    151–152
Respect for clients 134–135
Retirement
    case study, Charles Walters 14, 15,
        41–50
    preparation for 48–49
Role conflicts 19, 20, 152
Role models 87, 152
Role reversal 64

S

Self-awareness 116, 152
Self-efficacy 130, 152
    case study, Dorothy Atkins 119–126
Self-esteem
    components 32
    definition 152
    patient 28, 30, 134
    practitioner 15
Self-help groups 48
Self-image 31, 87, 152
Self-perception
    altered 73–74
    conflicts 31
    theory 152
Sexism 30
Sick role 13–14, 24, 45, 152
    case study, Charles Walters 14, 15,
        41–50
'Skiism' 55–56
Smoking
    cessation, case study, George Archer
        15, 137–145
    and coronary heart disease (CHD)
        140
    and diabetes 46, 138–140
    and menopause 30–31
    as stress-relief 27, 28
SMR *see* Standardized mortality rate
Social cognition models 42–43

Social constructionism 57
Social effects of partner loss 71
Social identity
  definition 153
  during adolescence 101, 102, 134
  following retirement 48–49
Social isolation 124–125
Social learning theory 57, 153
Social life
  client 81, 103
  practitioner 21
Social networks 120, 121–123
  case study, Dorothy Atkins
    119–126
  and individual behaviour 124
  influential characteristics 124
  morbidity and mortality rates
    122–123
Social perception theories 52
Social support, perceived/structural
  130
Social *vs* medical needs, case study,
  Margaret Knowles 18, 109–117
Society of Chiropodists and
  Podiatrists 24, 26
Socioeconomic status
  classification of occupations 78–79
  and health, case study, Bill Canning
    15, 77–84
  health inequalities 79–80, 82, 83,
    115, 139, 142
Somatic symptoms 73–74
Spina bifida 127, 128–129
  case study, Sophie Miller 127–136
Standardized mortality rate (SMR) 80
Stoicism 111, 112–114, 120
Stress
  and ageing 124–125
  and bereavement 72
  definition 153
  effects on health 72–74
  model 73
  in newly qualified podiatrists 19–21
  in retirement 49
Stress-reduction strategies 20–21
  smoking 27, 28
Stroke 61–62, 138
  case study, Sheetal Joshi 14, 61–66
Student podiatrists *see* Professional
  training
Supervision 20, 21
Susceptibility 29, 74
Synergy 31

T

Team roles 4–5
Team work 47–48
Theory of planned behaviour 44–45
Theory of reasoned action 42, 44–45
Therapeutic relationships 3–4, 13–15
  with adolescents 104, 134–135
  communication skills 15, 18, 32–35,
    82
  concordance 36, 38, 57, 58, 149
  establishing 35–38
  factors affecting 37
  influencing behavioural beliefs
    43–44
  power shift 36
  private practice *vs* health service 24
  typologies 24, 35–36
Therapeutic touch 34
Time management 20
Time pressures 19
Training
  'deviancy' 102
  excessive exercise 51, 53–54, 55–56,
    87–88, 103
  professional 2–5, 9, 13
Transient ischaemic attack (TIA) 62
Transtheoretical/Stages of Change
  Model 141–142, 145

U

Universal precautions 95–96, 98
Unpleasant sights and smells 116

V

Vulnerability 68, 72–73, 153

W

Weight gain 27, 31
Weight loss 103
Willingness to pay 80, 81–82
Workload 19
Written information 36